The Old Days are Back

Chair Yoga Exercises for Seniors Over 60 to Improve Stability and Posture

By

HNM Books

Legal Notice

Disclaimer Notice

This book is written and published independently. Please keep in mind that the material in this publication is solely for educational and entertaining purposes. All efforts have provided authentic, up-to-date, trustworthy, and comprehensive information. There are no express or implied assurances. The purpose of this book's material is to assist readers in having a better understanding of the subject matter. The activities, information, and exercises are provided solely for self-help information. This book is not intended to replace expert psychologists, legal, financial, or other guidance. If you require counseling, please get in touch with a qualified professional.

By reading this text, the reader accepts that the author will not be held liable for any damages, indirectly or directly, experienced due to the use of the information included herein, particularly, but not limited to, omissions, errors, or inaccuracies. As a reader, you are accountable for your decisions, actions, and consequences.

Contents

<u>Introduction</u>

By the time you are 60, you will have likely walked two million steps. You have probably experienced your fair share of illnesses or pain.

But I have a solution for you. It is Chair Yoga.

According to statistics, 14 million yogis in the USA are over 50, and 87% of them feel that yoga relieves their back pain boosting their well-being.

Apart from ageing is steadily slowing down. Many seniors have the rare opportunity to slow down in their everyday activities, far from the hectic pace of youth and middle age. Some seniors may need to move at a slower pace due to injuries or chronic pain, while others may just desire to be more deliberate in their daily activities. Fortunately, chair yoga can help seniors like you with restricted mobility to keep yourself active and adapt to the natural ageing process.

You can perform chair yoga while seated in a chair or using a chair as support. It is one of the more mild yoga types for seniors and offers routines at various levels of difficulty. So, if you feel apprehensive about exercise or have mobility issues, you can benefit from chair yoga because it is tailored for seniors.

My nana is 68 years old and lives alone. Let me tell you about her experience with chair yoga.

She did not have any severe pains or much difficulty moving around. However, I often used to get calls from her to come over and help her out around the house. Being a physiotherapist, I recommended she exercise to help improve her physical well-being and avoid any future mishaps. The thing about my nana is that she is very resistant to change. She would always brush my suggestion off or promise to talk about them later, but she never would.

One day my assistant took a call for me while I was in a meeting and explained that my nana had called an hour ago and that she needed me at the house. I called her back, and she would not return my calls. My office was an hour away from her home, and I rushed there, worried as fast as I could. When I entered, I saw nana lying on the floor. Turn out, she was sitting on the sofa and could not get up, so she wiggled her way out of the sofa to get to the phone but fell to the floor. Needless to say, there was no getting up from that. She lay there in pain for two hours! I told her it was enough.

After consultation with her doctor, I put her on chair yoga. She practised yoga at home for 4 months and now even goes out to the park every morning with her friends for a walk. I still get calls from her but only to come to eat her yummy pies.

Chair yoga includes helpful exercises, especially for pain relief and mobility issues for seniors, since you can adjust the sequences according to each person's level of competence, with a gentle and painless progression that gradually builds a senior's confidence. Seniors remain active and increase their strength and flexibility with these yoga poses without making major or full-range motions.

There is growing evidence that yoga therapies may improve older persons' functioning capacities. A chair yoga intervention with elderly persons over 80 has been shown to increase balance and walking speed, according to a study. A different study showed that older persons with Alzheimer's disease who participated in the "Fit Chair Yoga" program saw improvements in both physical and mental abilities.

The benefits of chair yoga are tremendous for senior citizens, including relaxing and stretching sore muscles, minimizing chronic pain, lowering stress levels, and enhancing circulation. Additionally, it reduces stress, assists in lowering blood pressure, safeguards joints, and improves strength and balance.

The short book "Chair Yoga Workout for Seniors over 60" focuses on helping seniors regain their independence and health through easy yoga poses with chair support that can be performed at home without equipment.

The book contains two sections, with the first introducing seniors to chair yoga, its benefits, requirements and precautions. It ends with helping you devise your own exercise plan according to your needs and ease.

The book's second section contains four chapters devoted to step-by-step yoga poses guidance for better flexibility, balance and stability, posture and boosting body strength. These chapters will also help you reduce back pain and muscle strain.

As I mentioned before, I am a physiotherapist with 9 years of professional experience. I deal with people of all ages daily, but most of my patients are seniors. My older patients find chair yoga the easiest way to improve their body health. They have claimed that independence and reducing body pain make them feel good mentally and reinforce a happy lifestyle. I have included the most effective yoga poses I personally suggest to my patients and have proven to work wonders for them, including my nana.

You must speak with your doctor before starting any new workout program and talk over any potential issues or adjustments that may be required.

Then we can get started on your wellness journey!

Chapter 1: Crash Course on Chair Yoga for Beginners

Sometimes in life, you must call on the strength you did not know you had. Losing mobility and independence, or living in a body that is constantly in pain, are challenges that might awaken the human spirit's inherent ability to fight pain and maintain confidence in what is in your potential. Yoga is the lifeline that ties us to our innate power for many who practice it.

A study on chair yoga and osteoarthritis was published in 2017 in The Journal of Geriatrics. Chair yoga was practised by those who were affected by this disease twice a week for 45 minutes each session. The eight-week experiment was conducted. Participants thereafter reported less pain, enhancements in daily activities, and improved walking speaking. A smaller study from 2012 and an earlier one from 2010 both discovered that chair yoga helped seniors feel less stressed and lowered their chance of falling. It is crucial to think about these findings. After all, falls among seniors are a major contributor to fatal and nonfatal injuries.

Although chair yoga research provides strong evidence, real-life examples are often much more compelling. So let me share two such stories.

Derek's Story

Derek's life took an unexpected turn at the age of 38. He was a construction manager, a father of two teenage boys, and a competitive runner. He was injured in an automobile accident that almost killed him and left him paralyzed from the chest down. Derek had to breathe through a tracheostomy tube for over two and a half years after spending a month in intensive care and the following nine months in rehabilitation. He learned how to use a wheelchair by using his upper body strength throughout rehabilitation. "Focus on your upper body, on what you have, and forget about the rest of your body," was his advice.

However, Derek had always loved being active and the athletic rush of basketball and running. Derek started going to chair yoga classes on a regular basis and saw that he was regaining his once lost sense of total body awareness. His yoga practice has completely changed him, giving him more independence by enhancing his balance and body confidence to the point that he can now get from his chair to his bed by himself.

Jack's Story

Jack, 56, woke up one morning five years ago with leg and back pain so severe he could hardly move. Although he had been battling it for months and attempting to control it with medicines, this was different. The doctor informed him that he had damaged cartilage in two of his lumbar vertebrae and would probably need surgery. Jack visited the hospital for an epidural two days later to manage the discomfort.

His daughter, who was driving, stopped the car on the way home, switched off the engine, and threatened to stop unless he agreed to accompany her to a yoga lesson. Jack claims that his daughter had good reason to be concerned about him. He never scheduled any time for exercise or self-care. He had three girls to raise, a difficult divorce to deal with, a demanding career as a manager at a technology company, and he also helped lead the local Hispanic Chamber of Commerce. He drank up to 10 caffeinated diet drinks daily to maintain vigour. He had gained 50 pounds. Jack added, "I could tell I couldn't keep it all together. It was frightful."

After two weeks, he attended a chair yoga class. His pain was reduced by yoga, which helped to strengthen his core and loosen his back. The best part was that it gave him the resiliency to handle his hectic lifestyle. Jack enrolled in a 200-hour teacher training course a few months later. After three months of training, he had shed the additional pounds, stopped taking the majority of his prescriptions, and generally felt happy. He has not required any other epidurals or back surgery since that time.

I have a feeling you can make your own inspiring story so let me introduce you to chair yoga fundamentals.

1.1 The "What" and "Why"

Even though being active as you age can help you avoid age-related problems, older people are more likely to suffer from strains, injuries, or joint pain. Yoga can help in this situation. Seniors who practice yoga can increase their muscle power and flexibility without running the danger of straining their muscles.

To thrive as we age, we must modify our routines and way of life. Exercise can be more challenging if you have sore muscles, joint discomfort, weariness, or other age-related issues. These worries often cause seniors to lead a sedentary and inactive lifestyle, which only makes matters worse. Fortunately, chair yoga is an inexpensive and simple form of exercise that has tremendous benefits for seniors.

It is never simple to trace the origins of yoga asana and styles. However, Lakshmi Voelker-Binder is thought to have coined the term "Chair Yoga" in the 1980s. For individuals with restricted mobility for whom a bit physical postures were no longer feasible, she started creating chair sequences and postures. It provides all the advantages of yoga without putting strain on the joints, supporting the body's weight, or worrying about balance for yogis who have physical and weight differences. However, the origins might lie with B. K. S. Iyengar, the yoga practitioner renowned for using props like stools and chairs.

Let me show you how it can improve your health immensely.

Increased Flexibility

Beyond just practising yoga, flexibility—the capacity to bend, twist, stretch, and move with ease—is essential. It enables you to carry out your obligations and partake in your favourite pastimes. Although some people believe that losing flexibility with age is inevitable, they are wrong. The saying " lose it or use it" is true when it comes to the human body. You may enhance your mobility and increase your range of motion at any age by gently pushing your body with chair yoga.

Reduced Pain

As researchers have repeatedly shown, reduced pain is one of the benefits of exercise. It is because exercise causes the body to release endorphins, a natural painkiller. You can manage your pain with the help of chair yoga as well. In other scenarios, pain and discomfort can be managed by gentle movement, deep breathing, and visualizing the pain leaving the body.

Improved Proprioception

Yoga involves fluidly shifting from one posture to another. Your proprioception is improved by changing poses. Proprioception: What is it? It is your capacity to precisely determine your body's location in space. Your coordination gets improved when your proprioception gets better. Additionally, your chance of falling is reduced.

Boosts Strength

Yoga poses make use of your muscles, which develops strength. Better balance brought on by increased strength can lower your risk of falling. Additionally, it can increase your body's resistance to injury. Your capacity to burn calories rises with increased muscle mass, which may also increase bone density and facilitate daily tasks.

Reduced Stress

Yoga naturally includes mindfulness. A form of moving meditation that encourages relaxation, eases tension and enhances mental clarity can be created by paying attention to your movement, breathing, and how your body is responding to the activity. Seated yoga, like other forms of exercise, has been shown to reduce anxiety and depression, boost confidence, and enhance mood.

Relieving Body Aches

Ageing is associated with a number of physical illnesses, particularly discomfort in the muscles and joints. With the use of specialized poses and stretches that reduce inflammation in tight and stiff muscles and joints, yoga is adaptive enough to meet these needs. Slow movements can reduce pain, and breathing exercises can help chronic pain sufferers learn to calm their brains and deal with any pain waves that may come. In other instances, yoga has helped older individuals wean themselves off of their dependence on painkillers.

Better Sleep

Chair yoga falls into the category of regular workout routines that are frequently linked to improved sleep. A more optimistic attitude on life, which in turn lessens stress and headaches and enhances sleep, has been linked to these mindful exercises, producing a mind-body experience.

Improved Balance and Coordination

Through changing poses, chair yoga helps your body become more spatially aware. Yoga teaches you to focus and use all the different areas of your body, making you feel closer to your physical self. You gradually get better coordination and balance training from doing this.

Boosts Muscle Power

It is a terrific approach to develop your muscles to practice chair yoga. This can lead to an improvement in flexibility, balance, and mobility. Building muscle also helps to keep your body from damage.

Improves Vascular Circulation

Adopting chair yoga improves the body's normal blood circulation. Yoga can enhance the balance of the body and the brain by increasing the amount of oxygenated blood sent to the fingers, toes, and brain.

Heart attacks and strokes are substantially less likely to occur as a result of better vascular circulation.

Inhibits Anxiety

Two parts of yoga that improve attention are breathing and movement patterns. This is a fantastic method to lessen some of the stress from daily life. You must meditate as part of the yoga practice, which can help you unwind and reduce any tension you may be experiencing.

Increased Spinal and Bone Health

Yoga is an organic weight-bearing activity. Consequently, it aids in evenly distributing your weight by helping you straighten your spine. This maintains the flexibility of your spinal discs and enhances posture. Additionally, it moves all 300 joints, boosting bone density and preventing osteoporosis.

Lowers Cholesterol

According to several research studies, seniors who regularly practised yoga had lower levels of bad cholesterol, lowering their risk of developing heart disease. It is due to the fact that yoga methods can assist in lowering stress, which in turn improves how well the body's organs work. Additionally, doing so can help you lose weight. Consequently, this combination lowers levels of harmful cholesterol and encourages healthier cardiac functions.

So, you see how chair yoga can help you! Chair yoga is a practical, affordable practice that does not need a lot of equipment or training. You only need a chair and a straightforward instruction manual to practice. You generally would not need a teacher because the exercises are straightforward, and you may complete them in the convenience of your own home. If help is required, a family member or caregiver can help. Let's get into the details of dos or don'ts for chair yoga.

1.2 The "Shoulds"

Understanding your limitations and not pushing yourself beyond what your body can tolerate is the most important step in developing a new fitness routine. If you have a previous disease that limits your mobility, you should especially seek a doctor's guidance on any moves you should avoid.

It is important to pay attention to how your body is positioned when doing yoga. Still, imagine that your body is in pain or has a limited range of motion. If so, you can adjust practically any stance to meet your needs. Remember that you are the best person to understand your body. So, whenever you do yoga, pay attention to your body. Here are a few straightforward modifications you may make to yoga poses. Try these tweaks whenever a pose hurts or feels like it is putting too much strain on the body. Your flexibility should increase as you perform this pose, and soon you will not require the change.

Remember that your body constantly changes. You might need to make a change today that you did not require yesterday, and vice versa. Always pay attention to your body and take note of any moves that produce discomfort or stress. If necessary, be ready to modify a movement. For instance, it is one thing to feel a stretch in a muscle you have not used in a while, but continuously using a muscle till it hurts might result in injury. Do not worry regarding your ability to stretch. Your ability to stretch more deeply will increase as you gain experience.

If you are hesitant to carry out the stretches recommended in this book, speak with your doctor.

Adjust the Angle

Imagine that you are performing standard standing yoga positions. If that is the case, you can benefit from spreading your legs out slightly wider than hip-width apart to relieve strain on your lower back. That can entail placing your feet slightly to the side rather than directly in front of you when performing chair exercises, for instance.

Reduce the Depth

Lift your arms with the best effort you can make if you cannot lift them over your head. It is also acceptable if you are unable to bend forward and touch your toes. Lift your hands to shoulder height as opposed to above your head. Lift your arms as high as you can while maintaining a full breath during the pose. You will notice that you have become more flexible as you continue to practice yoga. You will find it simpler to extend your stretches.

Add a Prop

Use a yoga block, cushion, or even a stack of books to prop up your feet if it is not possible to put them on the floor so that your legs are in the right posture. Injury can result from incorrect body positioning. A yoga strap, belt, or towel can be utilized as additional props to increase the stretch in your legs during exercises like the hamstring stretch.

A pillow can be helpful to include. Instead of a soft armchair, a durable kitchen chair would be the best choice for chair yoga. For some people, this could be uncomfortable. Your hips can be raised using a small pillow or towel to relieve some pressure and discomfort. Additionally, some postures, such as the Seated Forward Fold, may make it uncomfortable to maintain a forward bend. Place a cushion or towel on your lap and concentrate on leaning forward into this prop in this situation.

Make an Exercise Plan

Consider creating an exercise plan once you have given some of the exercises in this book a try and after you have decided what your fitness objectives are. Following a plan, you may monitor your development as you increase your flexibility and fitness. Assessing your level of fitness honestly is the first step. The workouts recommended in this book would not get you sweating as aerobic exercises will. However, they might put some strain on muscles that are not used frequently. Start small, then gradually expand on your idea.

Set aside sometime each day or each week to do chair yoga. If you can do this on a regular basis, your strategy will be a lot easier to follow. Regular practice of the stretches and exercises will also result in significantly longer-lasting effects.

Consider mixing up your workouts. Consider stretching your upper body one day and working out your lower body the next. This will lessen the risk of developing muscular tiredness. You can use the following as a template for creating your own exercise plan by using the example provided below:

Sunday

Breathing Exercises

and

10-Minute Gentle Yoga

Monday

Upper Body Routine

Tuesday

Neck and Shoulders Routine

Wednesday

Hips and Legs Routine

Thursday

Arm Focused Routine

Friday

Full Body Workout

Saturday

Pick Your Favorite

or

Work on a Specific Issue

Yoga may be practiced daily and is a fantastic method to keep your body healthy. Regular yoga practitioners can also anticipate improvements in their energy, flexibility, and mobility—all of which are crucial for seniors. In addition to enhancing mood and reducing sadness, yoga has also been shown to promote relaxation and mental clarity. Regular yoga practice can help to calm the mind and improve attention. Even older adults who are beginning to show signs of dementia have indicated that daily meditation and yoga practice help to decrease their symptoms.

Even older adults who are beginning to show signs of dementia have indicated that daily meditation and yoga practice help to decrease their symptoms. It is time to begin your yoga practice now that you are more knowledgeable about what chair yoga is and who it is intended for. Each section will concentrate on a particular body part or set of muscles. To design a program perfectly tailored to your needs, either follow the exercises exactly as they are written out or alter the order. Yoga techniques should be varied and alternated frequently to ensure that all muscle groups are being exercised during practice.

1.3 Getting Started

Yoga is a mind-body discipline that combines physical postures, meditation, and breath exercises. Before getting started, I want to introduce you to some breath work. While seated in a chair, one can perform a variety of breathing exercises. You can try these two separate exercises:

Exercise 1

1. This exercise is a wonderful approach to begin your practice because it helps to soothe the nervous system.
1. Put your feet on the ground firmly and sit up straight to begin this exercise.
1. Lie on your stomach with one hand and your chest with the other.
1. Breathe in slowly via your nose, filling your chest and stomach first.
1. Exhale gently through your nostrils, starting with your stomach and working your way up to your chest.
1. Repeat this breath time 3 times.

Exercise 2

This exercise can help you improve concentration and mental clarity.

1. Place both feet flat on the floor and sit up straight in your chair to perform this exercise.
2. Put your right hand in front of you and use your thumb to cover your right nostril. Breathe in deeply while slowly opening your left nostril.

3. Then, open your right nose and close your left nostril with your finger.

4. Slowly exhale by your right nostril.

5. Once more, breathe in through your right nostril, then seal it with your thumb and exhale through your left.

6. Use your left nostril to breathe out.

7. Follow the steps three to five times.

You can practice these two or any other favorite breathing exercise you have before performing yoga poses to help your mind relax and focus. The next chapters will focus on your issues one by one with detailed chair yoga exercises paired with illustrations.

Chapter 2:Regain Balance and Stability for Your Independence

Maintaining appropriate balance, gait, and range of motion is essential for the health and well-being of active older persons. Muscle mass and metabolism decline with age, and sedentary seniors frequently experience balance issues. Active seniors who practice balance exercises are usually better able to respond to daily demands and are less likely to fall.

As per CDC, the Centers for Disease Control and Prevention, one-third of Americans over 65 will fall at some point in the year. Balance training is crucial at this stage of life because falls are the second most common cause of brain and spinal cord injuries in later years.

Yoga is a useful method for improving balance, and individuals who cannot attend regular courses can still carry out many exercises with the assistance of a chair. The best aspects of flexibility and balance training are combined in chair yoga poses. The following chair yoga sequences use both static and dynamic forms of balance to enhance daily life activities.

2.1 Seated Mountain Pose

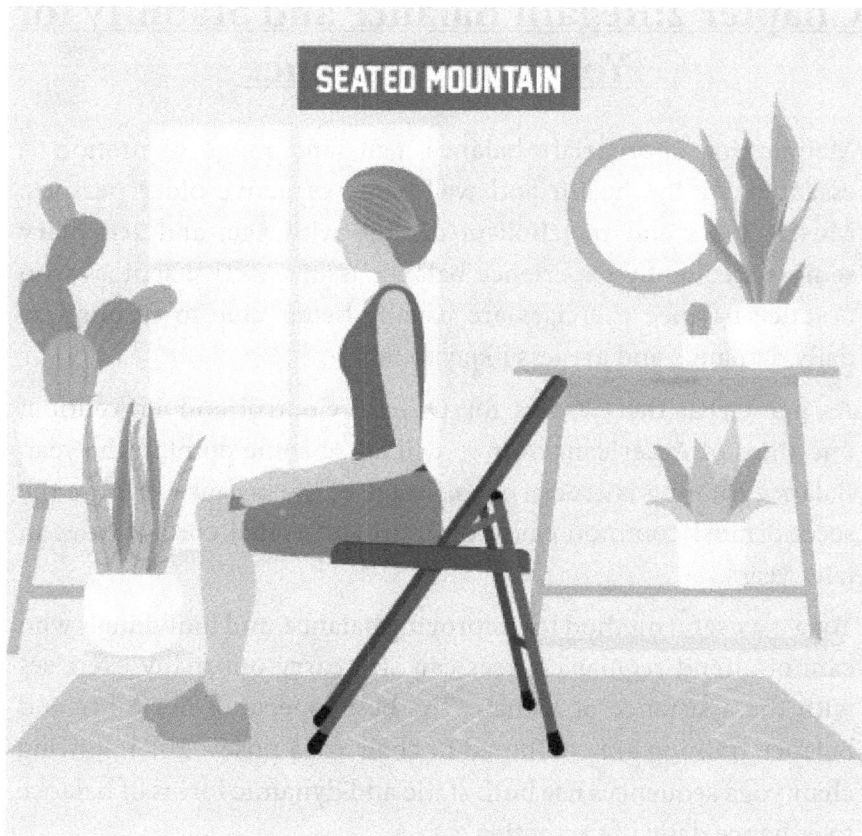

It is often used to reset and balance the body at the beginning of yoga practice and in between poses, the mountain position is also known as "samasthiti," which means "equal standing."

1. Place yourself on the chair's edge.

2. Your ankles should be immediately under your knees as you place your feet on the ground while bending both knees.

3. Put your feet firmly on the ground. Feel the center of your heel, your little toe mound, and your big toe mound all pressing equally hard into the floor.

4. As you firmly plant your feet, root your sitting bones into the chair's seat. Keep an eye out to see whether this tying down gives you a feeling of grounding.

5. Start growing upward from the roots you've established beneath you, up through your belly, pelvis, spine, and all the way to the top of your head.

6. During this rising up and descending, move your pelvis a few times forward and backward (first tipping forward on your sitting bones, then back), then find a neutral position in the center. The front rim of the pelvis would not be leaning forward or back when in neutral. Your right and left sitting bones will support the same amount of your weight.

7. The spine should also be in a neutral posture, with the lower back's natural inward curve at the lumbar spine, the middle and upper back's small outward curvature at the thoracic spine, and the neck's natural inward curve at the cervical spine (neck).

8. Then, with your chin parallel to the ground, the crown of your head rising toward the sky, and your gaze toward the horizon, bring your head into neutral by moving it squarely above your spine.

2.2 Seated Forward Bend

For this exercise, follow these steps:

1. Taking a deep breath, fold your legs over in the Seated Mountain pose, stretching your spine as you do so. Begin with your hands on your thighs and move them down your legs as you bend, or keep them at your sides as you work toward putting your torso on your thighs to provide a little extra support.

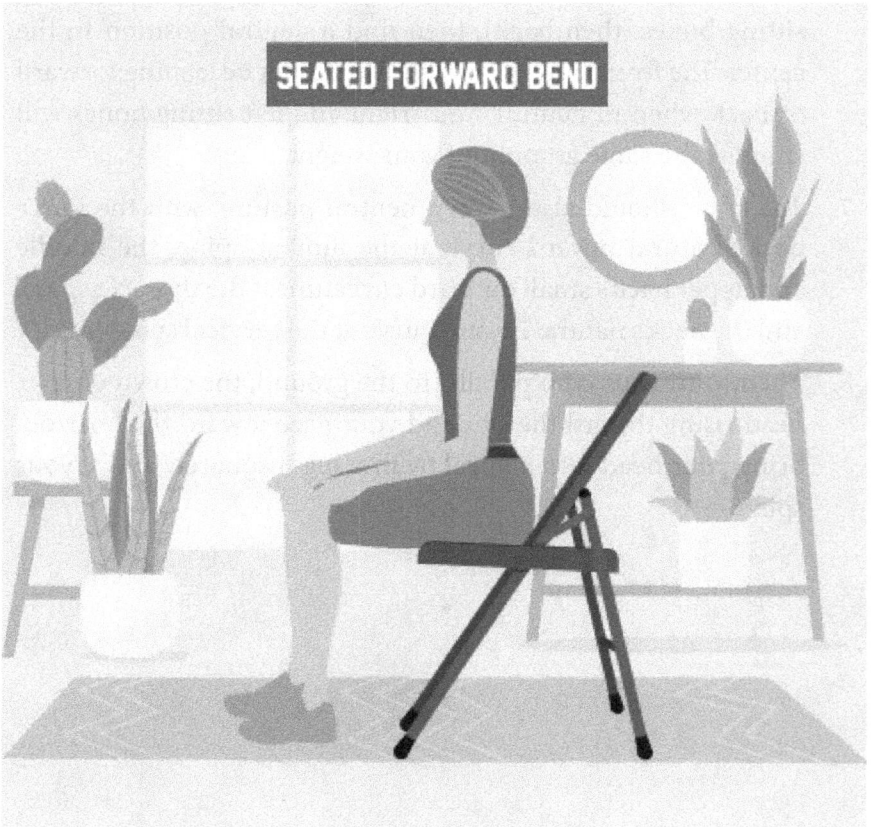

SEATED FORWARD BEND

3. In this position, inhale steadily for five breaths minimum. It slowly stretches and extends your back muscles as well as massages your intestines, which helps digestion.

4. When you are ready, take a breath and raise your torso back to

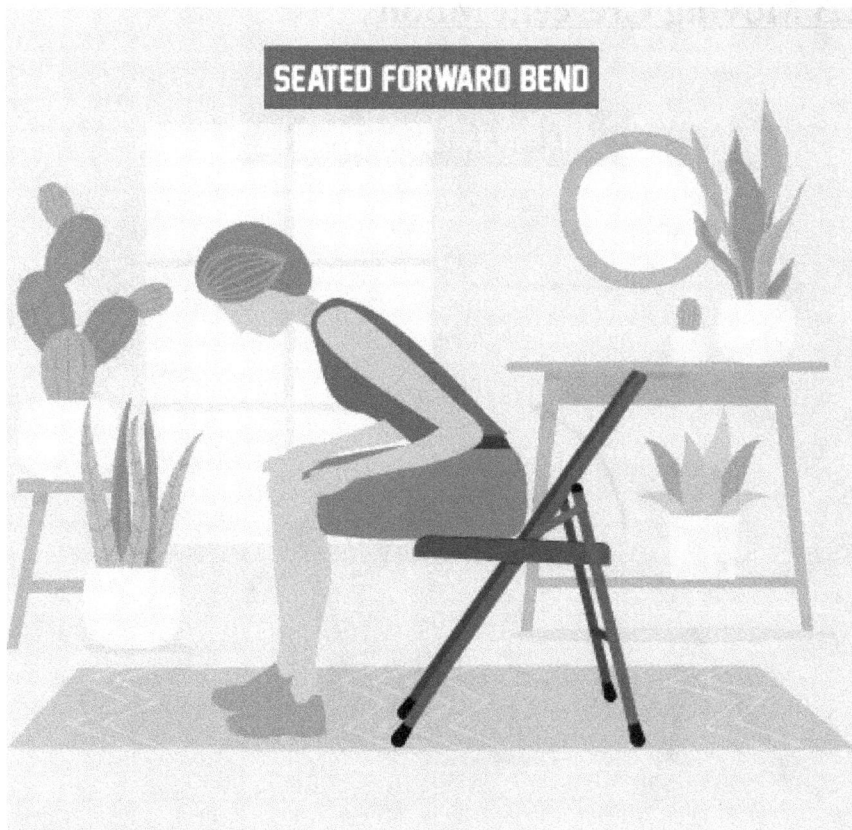

SEATED FORWARD BEND

its upright position.

2.3 Moving Crescent Moon

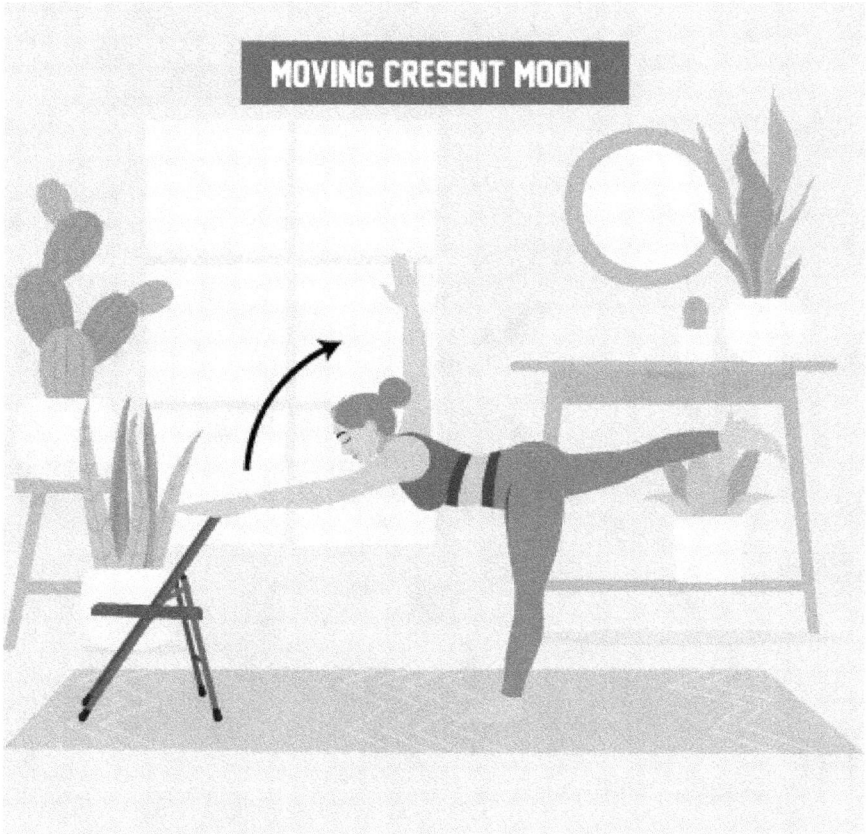

This exercise will help you improve your transitional balance. Here are the steps for it:

1. Stand behind the chair with your hands on the back of the seat.

2. Lifting the left heel off the ground, extend the left hand upward and move your weight to the right leg.

3. The motion resembles a side stretch.

4. Place both hands on the chair while moving the feet back to the middle.

5. Lifting the right heel off the ground while extending the right arm upward and stretching toward the left.

6. Continue moving in a side-to-side motion.

You can make this exercise easier by carrying out the steps while seated.

2.4 Eagle Arms

As your shoulder joint is stabilized and flexed in this pose, your shoulders and upper back are relaxed.

1. As you inhale, extend your arms out to the sides. Take a breath.

2. Swing your right arm beneath your left and grip your shoulders

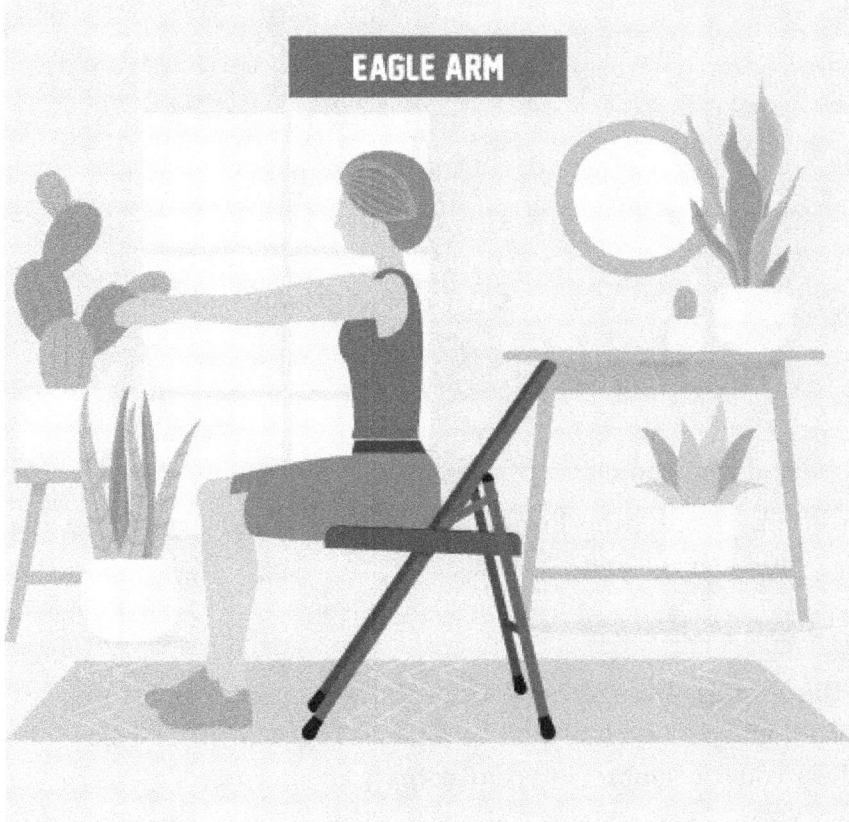

3. If your shoulders are flexible enough, you may let go of your grasp and keep hugging your forearms until your right fingers are resting in your left palm.

4. Lift your elbows a couple of inches higher while inhaling.

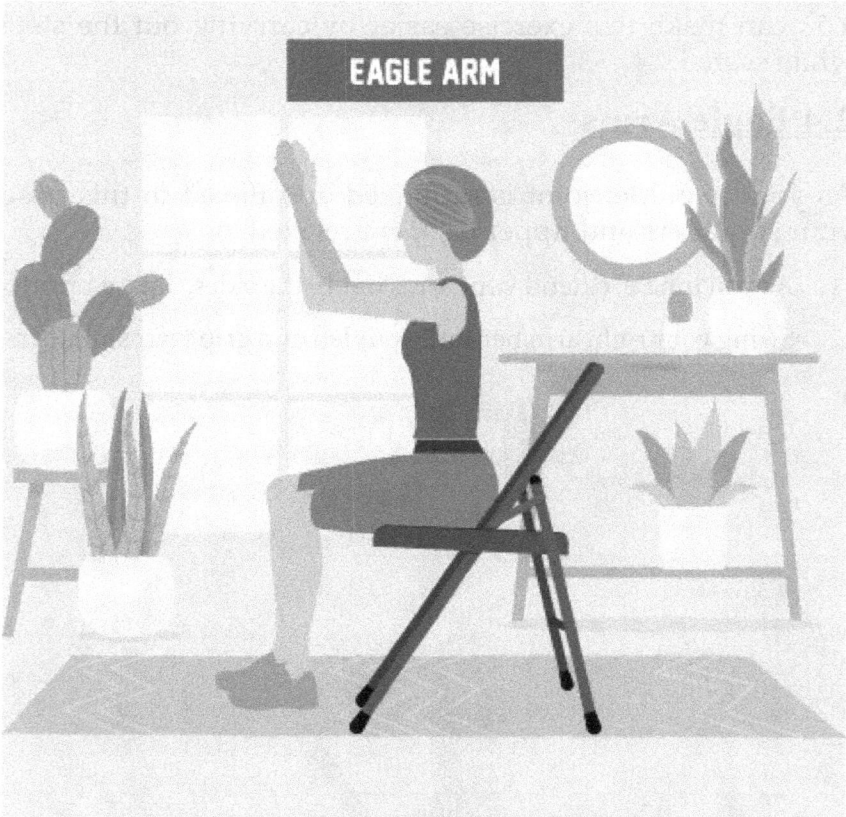

EAGLE ARM

5. Roll your shoulders away from your ears while exhaling.

6. Take a few deep breaths and, if you would like, repeat the shoulder roll and elbow raise.

2.5 Knee Raises

This exercise strengthens your thighs and hip flexors. Set up your workout space with a chair or a table. The steps listed below can help you start improving your stability and balance:

1. Put yourself behind or next to the chair.

2. Place your left hand on the back of the chair. Bend your left knee a little and balance on your left leg.

3. Keep your eyes glued to whatever is in front of you. Inhale deeply, and then exhale slowly.

4. As you exhale, move your right leg and bend it toward your chest. Avoid bending at the waist or the hips while performing this balance exercise.

5. Holding onto the chair, take a deep breath and elevate your knee to the count of one to three.

6. Exhale while lowering your leg back to the ground.

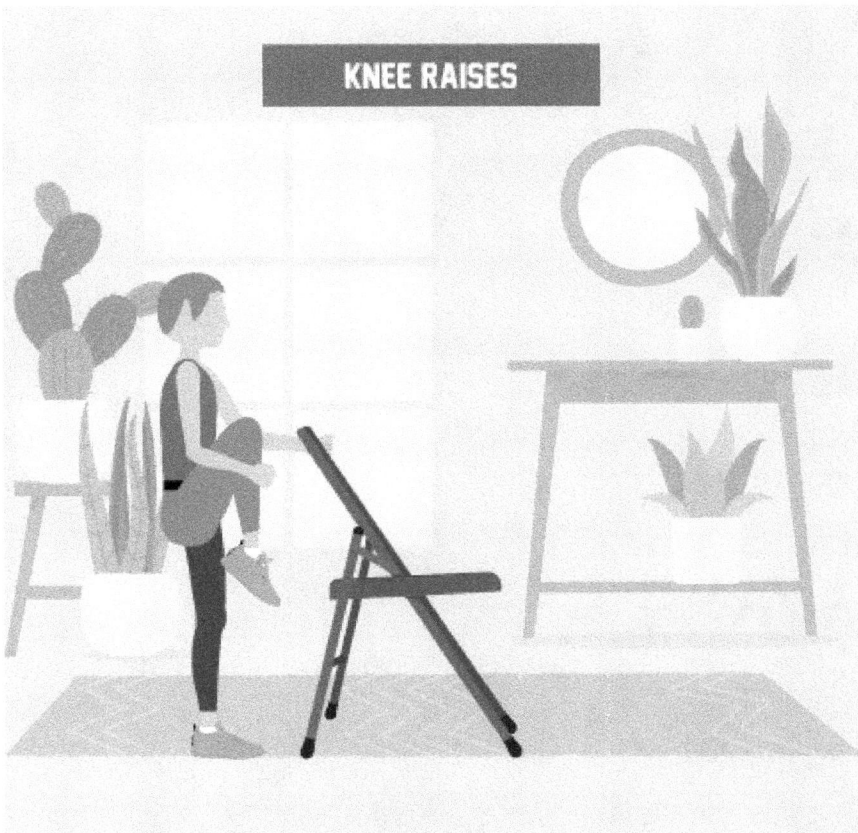

KNEE RAISES

7. Before switching legs, repeat this process several times.

Here are some advice and safety suggestions for you:

√ Simply dropping your legs down will give zero benefits to the exercise. Slowly reposition them in the beginning position.

√   Keep your knees bent if you are not yet comfortable with this exercise. The lower back is a lot stressed, and the hip flexors are worked more than the abdominals when the legs are stretched instead of bent at the knees. As your hips get stronger over time, you can expand your knees for a harder workout.

√   This exercise will require more momentum than muscle to execute if you move swiftly or swing your legs up and down.

2.6 Leg Raises

This exercise will concentrate on your core muscles, which include your thighs and hip flexors. Maintaining core stability can prevent injuries and falls. Leg lifts also tone your bottom and lower back. The directions for back and side leg lifts are as follows:

Back Leg Raises

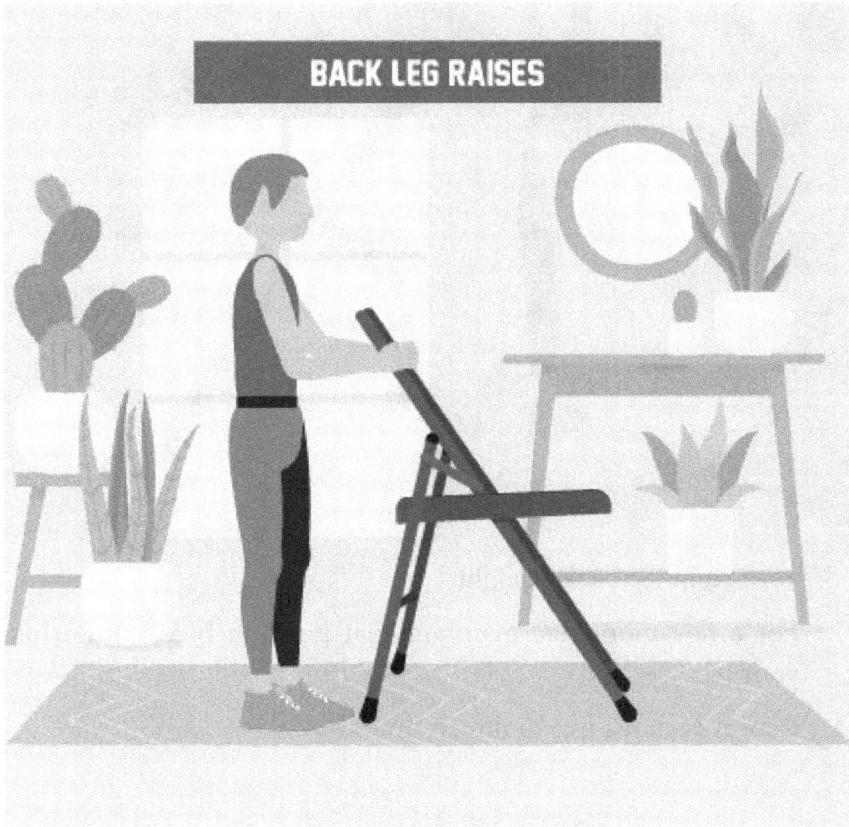

1. Stand behind a chair

2. Do not flex your knees or point your toes as you slowly raise

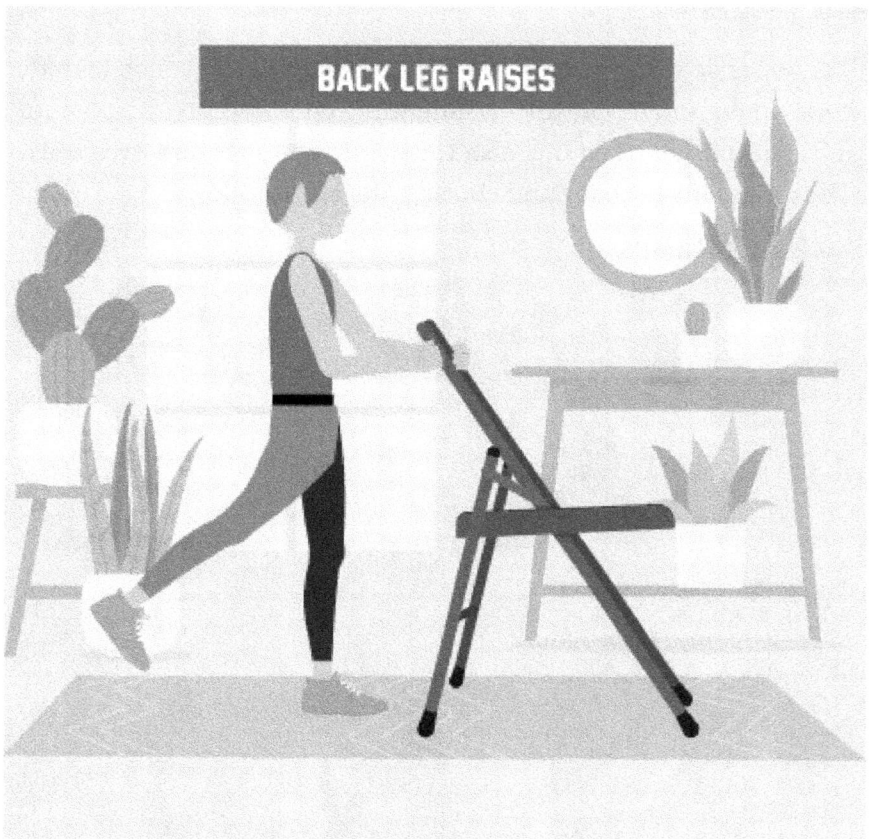

your right leg back straight.

3. For a few moments, maintain that position before lowering your leg.

4. Repeat each leg five to fifteen times.

Side Leg Raises

1. Take a position with your back straight behind or next to the

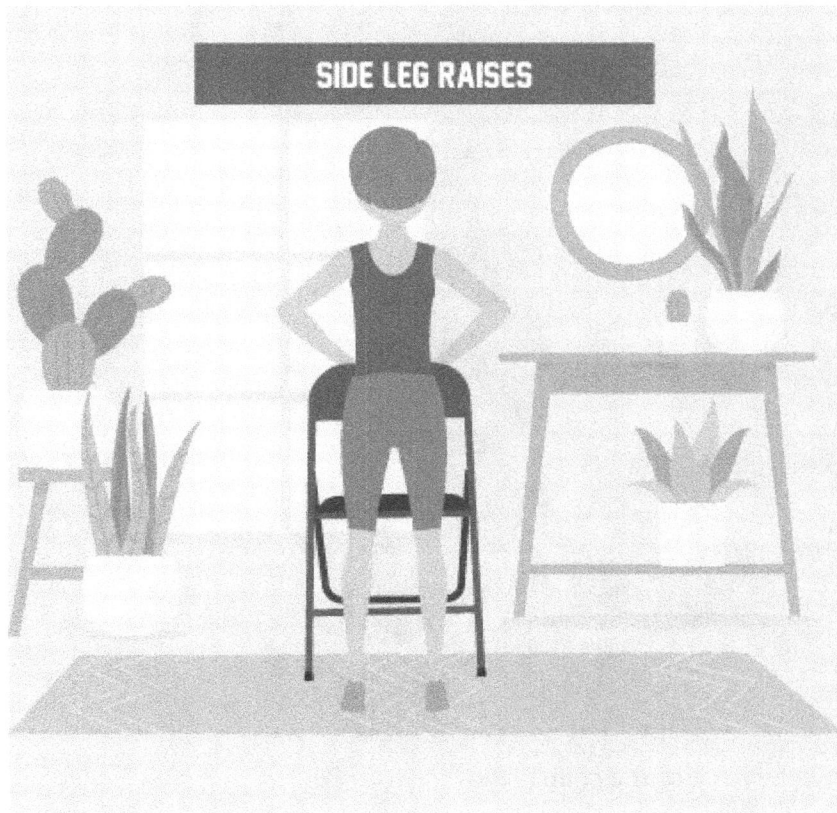

   chair.
2. Place your feet slightly apart and level with the ground. Grab

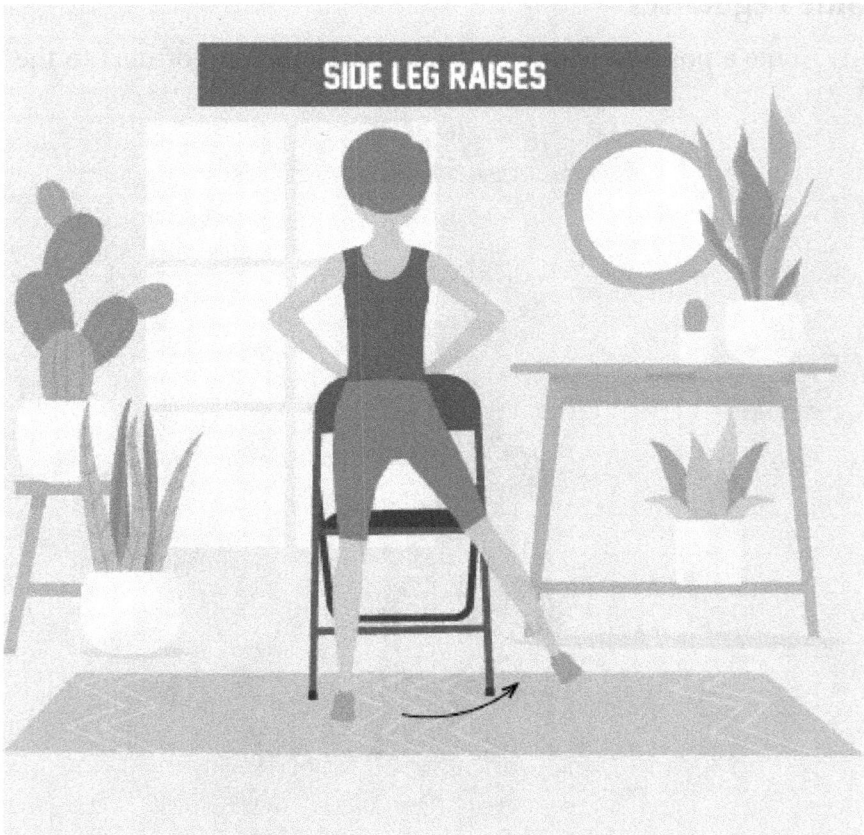

the back of the chair.

3. Exhale deeply and slowly lift your right leg 6 to 12 inches off the floor and to the side. Keep your body in a straight posture

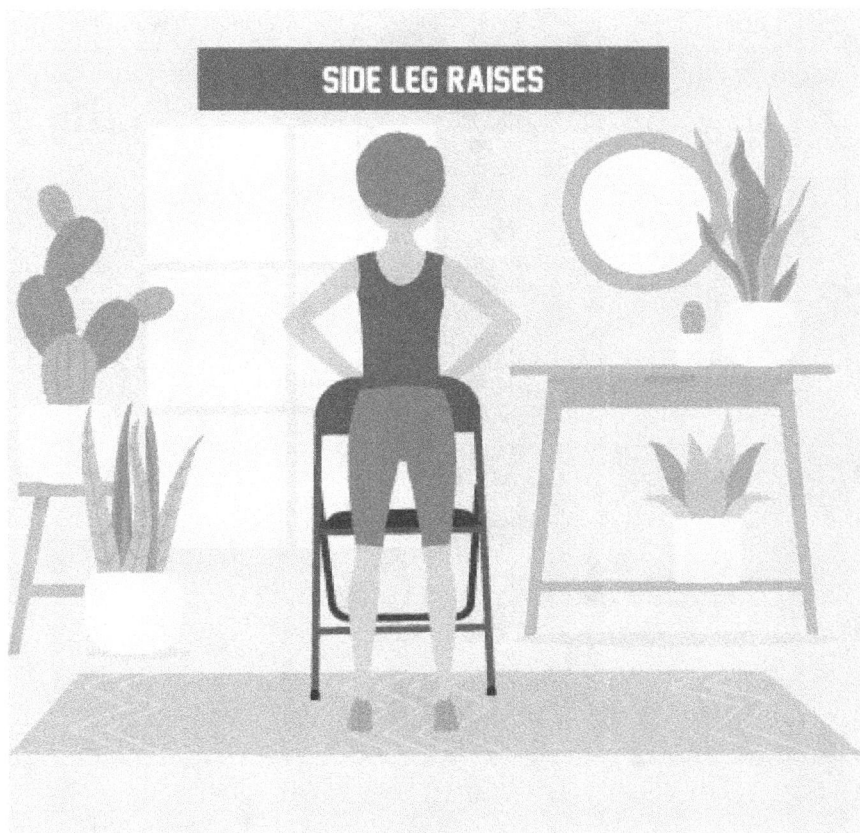

with your toes pointed forward.

4. Hold this position for a few seconds while taking a few deep

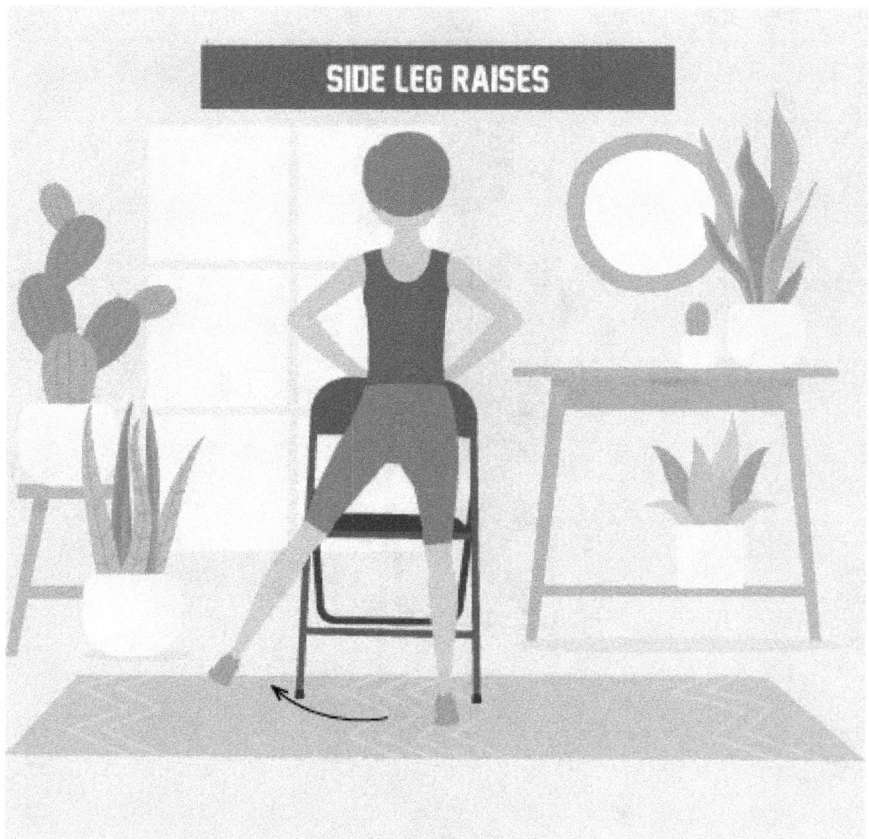

breaths. As you breathe, return to the starting posture.

5. Repeat a few times on one side before switching to the other leg.

2.7 Triangle

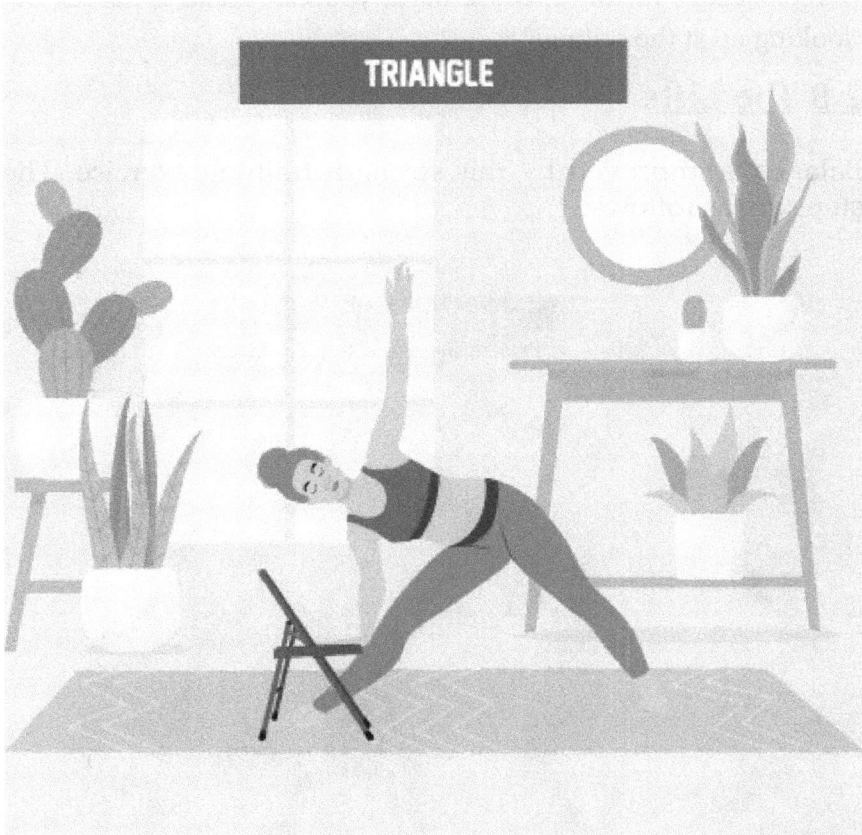

This yoga pose enhances balance in a unilateral stance. Here's how you can do it:

1. Step three to four feet away from a chair while standing sideways.

2. Turn the foot that is furthest away from the chair 45 degrees, then point the other foot's toes in the direction of the chair.

3. As you inhale, bring your arms to shoulder level.

4. Depending on your level of flexibility, exhale as you bring the arm that is closest to the chair to rest on the seat or back.

5. Keep holding and repeat on the other side.

As you adapt to this exercise hard, you can make it harder by looking up at the ceiling.

2.8 Toe Lifts

Balance is improved by this strength training exercise. The steps are as follows:

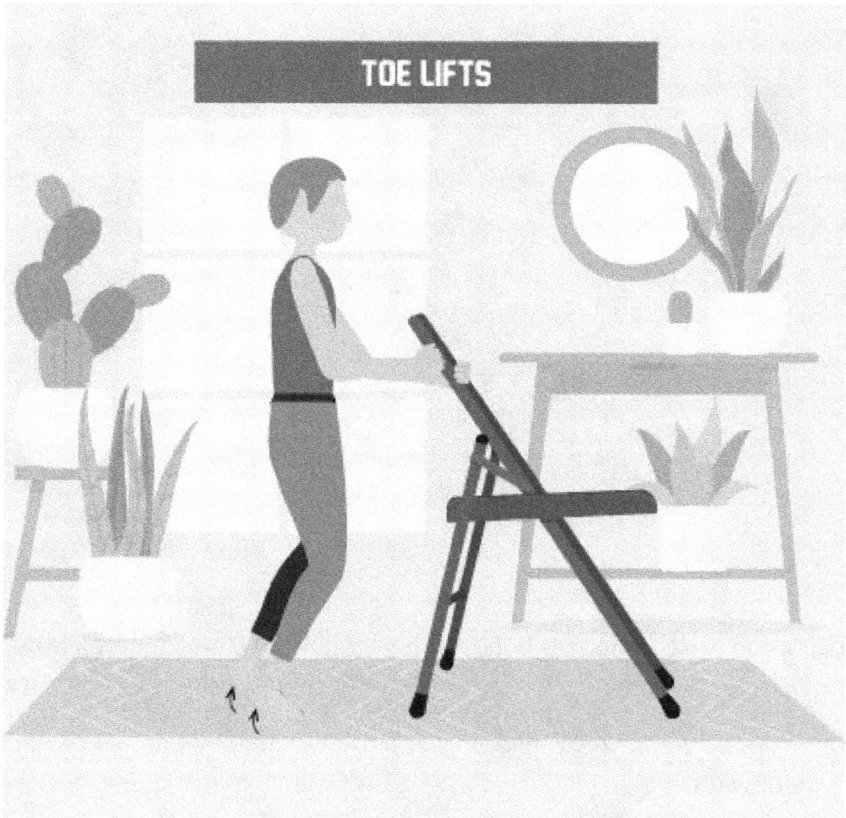

1. Stand up straight and cross your arms in front of your chest.

2. Raise yourself as much as you can using your toes.

3. Next, gradually lower yourself.

4. Avoid leaning too far forward at the counter or in your chair.

5. 20 times, lift your toes, then lower yourself.

2.9 Sit to Stand

For this one, you will need a chair that is appropriate for you. A kitchen chair is the ideal seating option (not a stool height). Sitting and standing help build your leg muscles and enhance your balance, even though it does not seem like exercise. A wonderful objective is to perform this workout three to four times weekly. Here are the instructions:

1. First, sit in the chair. Ensure that you are sitting on the chair's front edge rather than all the way back.

2. After taking a deep breath, slowly move by contracting your leg muscles. Hold on to the chair for support as you lean your

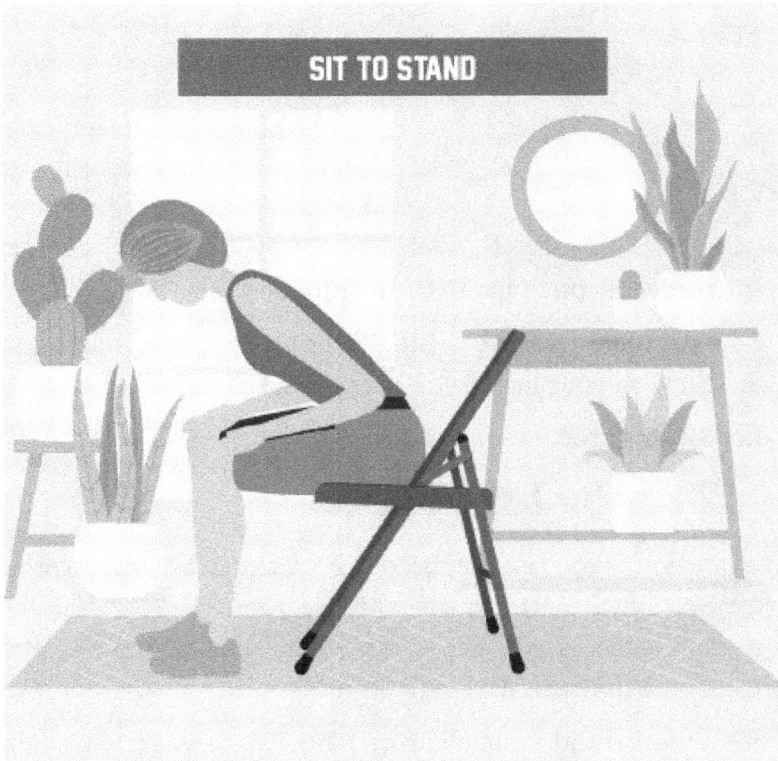

SIT TO STAND

chest forward slightly.

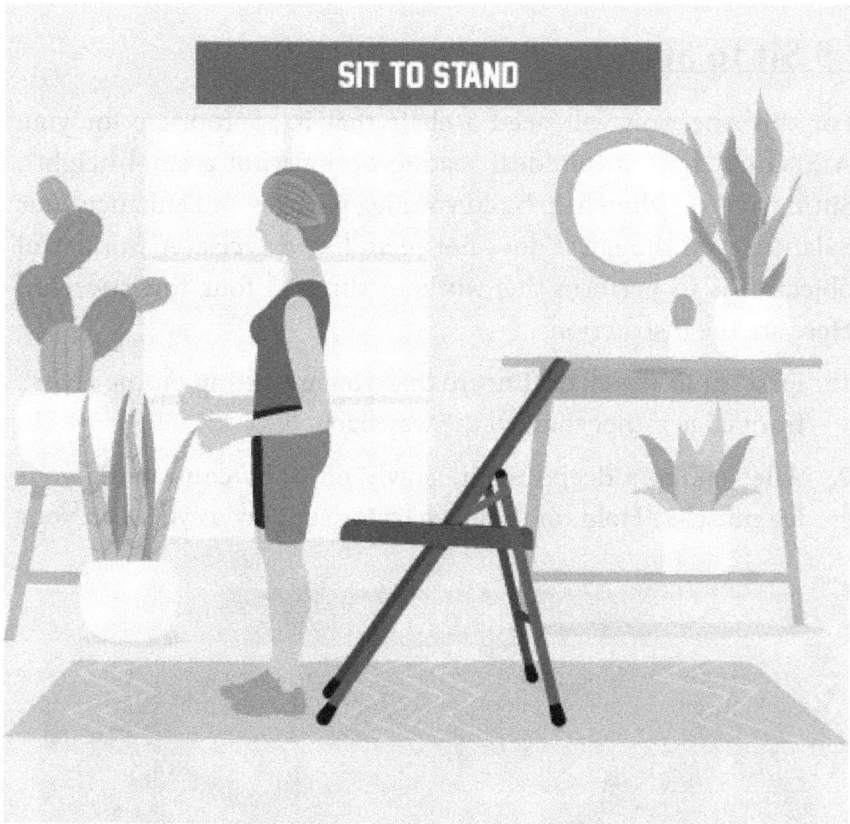

SIT TO STAND

3. Inhale deeply once again, then straighten your body.

4. As you exhale, lean over a little and sit back down, making sure the backs of your legs are resting on the chair legs.

5. Repeat this process several times.

2.10 Chair Hip Extensions

Hip extension is the last exercise in the series of balance exercises for seniors. Try to perform this exercise a few times a week. Add a few more reps as you get stronger, and consider doing these exercises on a different day. Let's begin:

1. Standing behind your chair or table, space your feet slightly apart on the ground.

2. Your feet should be spaced apart at shoulder width or slightly less.

3. Step back from the chair while maintaining a straight back.

4. Slowly raise one leg back while keeping the knee and leg

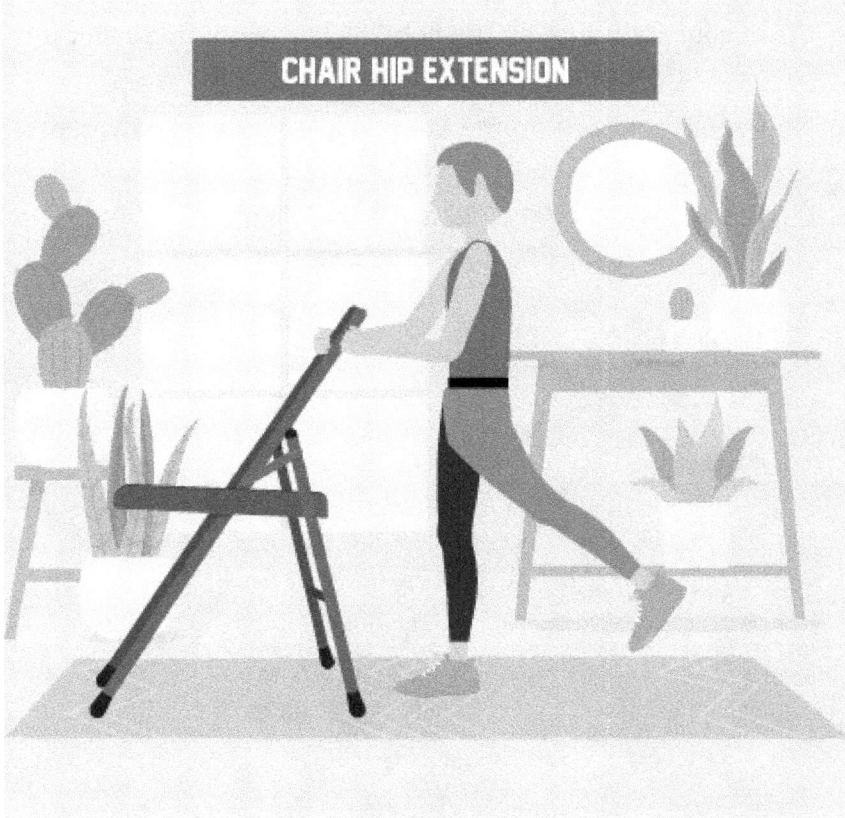

CHAIR HIP EXTENSION

straight. As you carry out this motion, maintain a straight back.

5. Hold the stance for a brief moment before carefully bringing your leg back to its starting position.

6. Before switching legs, repeat this process 10 to 15 times.

2.11 Standing on One Foot

This exercise helps you maintain your balance and increase your strength by working on your lower body muscles. Let's begin:

1. Take a light grip on the back of a sturdy chair.

2. Take your right foot off the floor. Slowly count up to ten. It is not a good idea to let oneself tilt to the left.

3. Put your foot back on the floor. When you are ready, repeat

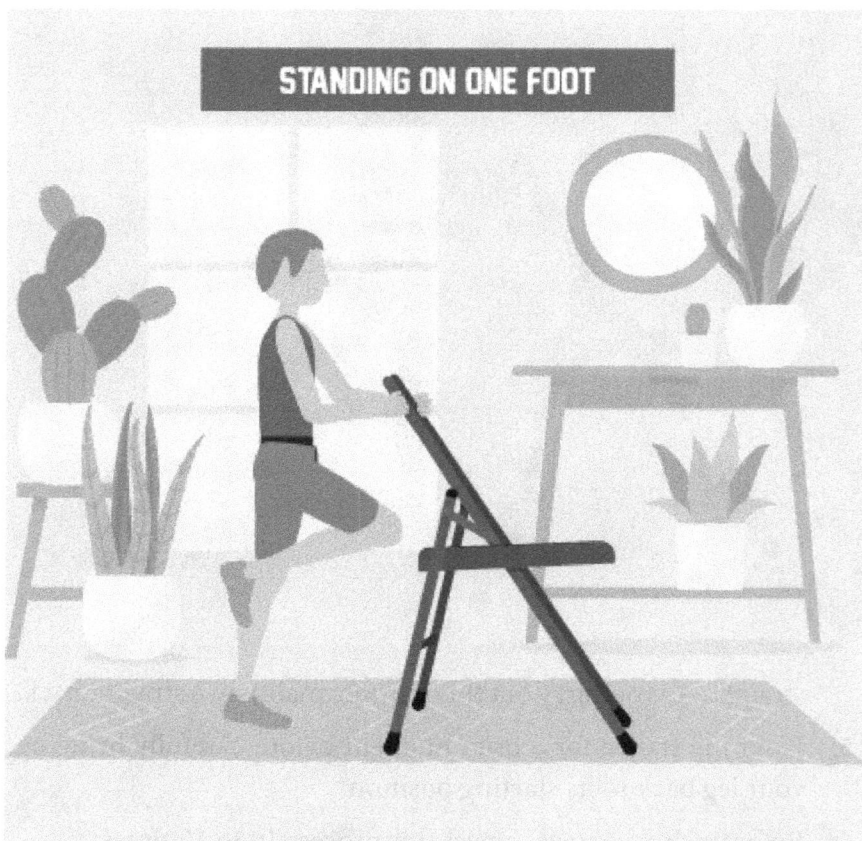

STANDING ON ONE FOOT

thesame with your second foot.

4. Every day, add 5 to 10 seconds to the time you spend balancing on each foot until you can do it for 30 seconds on each side with ease.

5. At this point, you can try to balance yourself without clinging to the chair. Start by giving each foot a 10-second hold while keeping your back to it in case you need to let your hands down. Once you can stand on each foot for a minute, extend your periods of balance.

6. By raising your legs higher or lifting your right arm above your head while lifting your left foot, and vice versa, you can make it harder for yourself.

2.12 Clock Reach

Clock reach might help you balance better when standing still. Along with strengthening your hip and ankle muscles, it also increases the range of motion in your shoulders and upper body.

1. Take a seat.

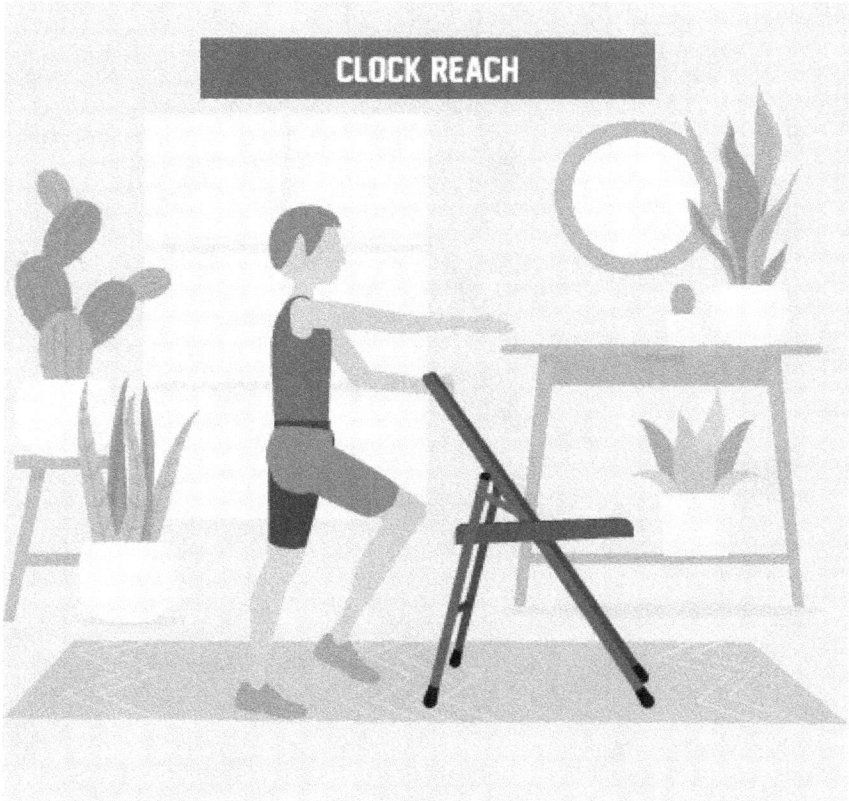

2. Think of a clock with hours 12 and 6 on either side of you.

3. On your left leg, raise your right arm to the hour mark.

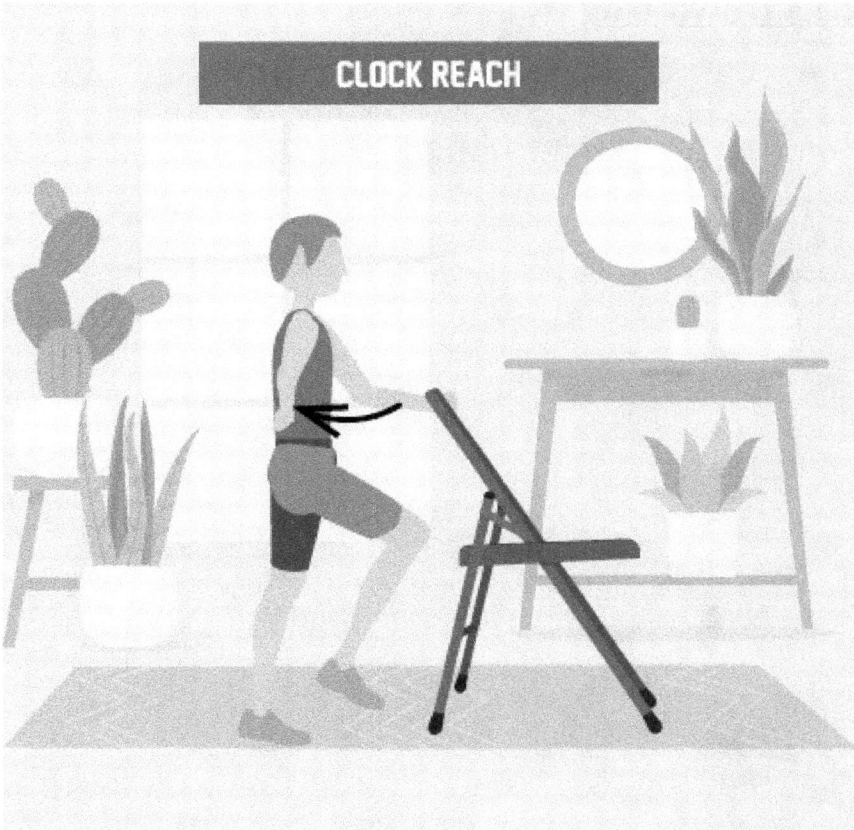

CLOCK REACH

4. Reach 3 and then 6 o'clock.

5. Repeat on the other side while standing on your right leg.

Following are some advice and safety measures for this exercise:

√ Raise your chest, adopt a powerful stance, and keep your eyes fixed on one thing at eye level.

√ Reach out as far as you are comfortable doing.

√ If reaching 6 o'clock is uncomfortable, stop at 3 o'clock.

2.13 Down Dog

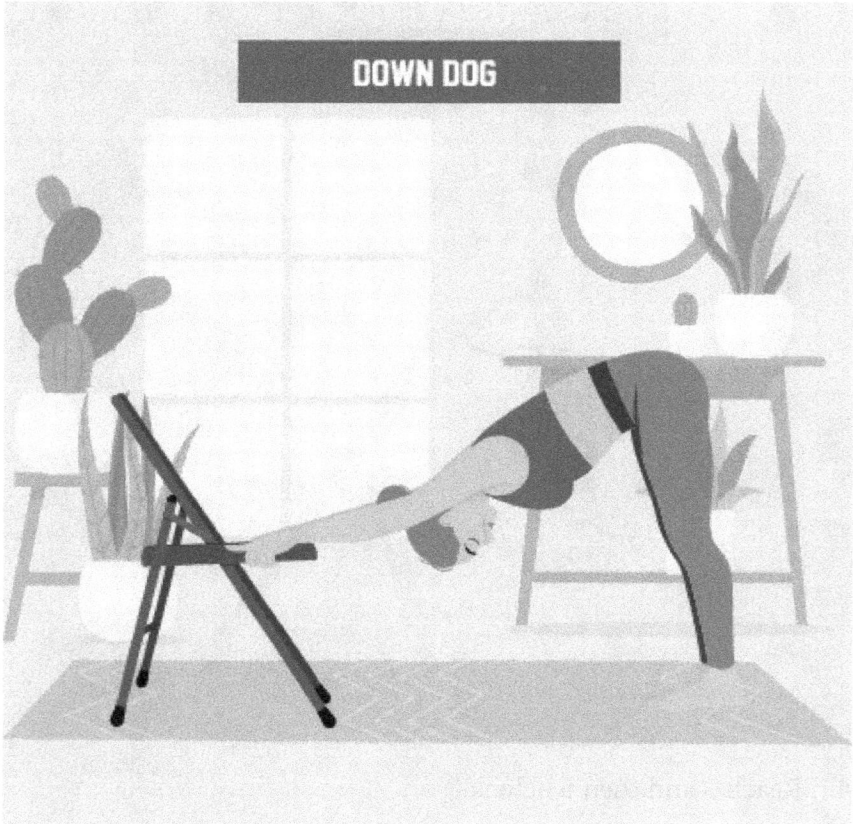

This exercise increases stability when inverted (head below the hips.) Here are the steps you need to take:

1. Stand with your back to the chair's base.

2. Raise your arms in the air as you inhale.

3. Put your hands on the chair's base as you exhale (bend knees if needed).

4. Lift the hips and slowly walk your feet back until you are in the down-dog position.

5. To exit the position, carefully move forward with your feet

until your body is folded forward.

6.   Move the body up one vertebra at a time to get back to standing.

You can put your hands on the chair's back to make this exercise easier.

These exercises will help you improve your balance so you can move around without dependence.

Chapter 3: Improve Your Posture and Reduce Muscle Strain

According to studies, practising yoga can correct hunched-over posture and even reverse the dowager's hump, a condition associated with ageing that affects posture. Our posture is a crucial aspect of health that does not always receive the attention it needs. Your posture affects how your spine is aligned, affecting how healthy your body is overall. Since the spine serves as the main conduit for the nervous system, a healthy spine ensures that the nervous system's pathways are strong and clear and that vital energy may flow through them freely to maximize vitality and well-being.

New research shows that maintaining good posture is crucial to living a long and healthy life.

Here are the yoga poses for posture and muscle strain.

3.1 Seated Gentle Backbend

Our thoracic and cervical spines, which make up our upper and midback, continue to bend forward as we age. Instead of being our "lazy" posture, it has the potential to become our "regular" posture. This strains the muscles in the back and contributes to the hunch we typically associate with getting older. This simple backbend will ease your tension.

Numerous health advantages of backbends improve your physical and emotional well-being. Physically, they support you in avoiding hunching forward or compromising your alignment and posture during regular activities. Gravitational stresses, excessive movement, and sedentary situations can all lead to misalignments and pain in the body. A fantastic method to realign your body is to do backbends.

Backbends are good for your chest, hips, shoulders, and back. By lengthening your spine, enhancing flexibility, and enhancing mobility, they assist in promoting good posture. Additionally, they help to relieve stress, stiffness, and discomfort.

Backbends' energetic qualities also warm and stimulate your body, which helps to relieve fatigue. In fact, because they can make it harder to fall asleep, strong backbends should be avoided right before bed. The steps are as follows:

1. Starting from a seated position with your feet flat on the floor, move your hands towards lower back with your fingers pointing down and put your thumbs on the hips in the direction of your

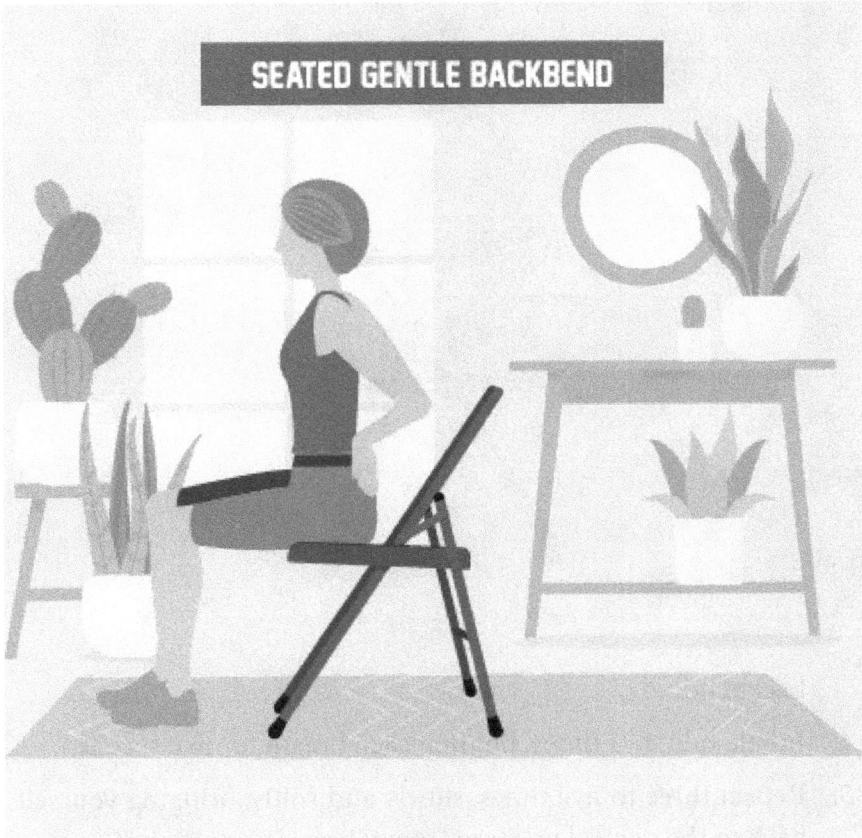

SEATED GENTLE BACKBEND

front body.

2. Inhale while firmly pressing your hands into your lower back and hips.

3. As you exhale, gently bend your spine, starting with your head. You do not want your head to sag too far back, so keep that in mind. A wise, gentle location to begin is with your chin tilted up and facing the ceiling as you do want to start with the cervical spine. Up to the mid-spine should be bent during the

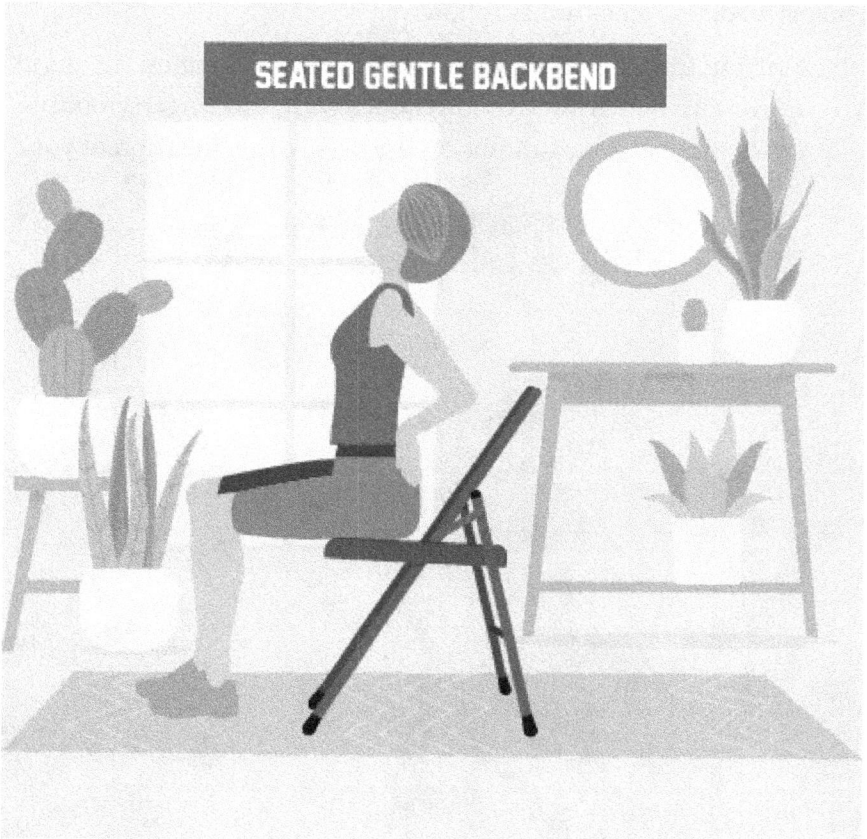

SEATED GENTLE BACKBEND

backbend.

4. Inhale fully five times, holding each breath for five seconds.

5. Repeat three to five times, slowly and softly, bringing yourself back to the neutral position from where you started.

Here are some safety measures and advice:

√ In order to benefit the most from backbends, they should be performed carefully and with mindfulness. Always warm your body before a backbend, and cool down afterwards. In addition to warming up your spine, perform exercises that target your upper body, hips, and thighs.

√ Do not hold challenging poses for too long, as well. To spend more time in the stance, you can hold it for a shorter amount of time and repeat it a couple of times. Take some time to thoroughly recover in between reps.

√ To prevent injury, do no more than three backbends in a row.

√ Never push yourself or stretch yourself into a position, and if you start to feel pain, cease right away. If you have neck pain, relax your neck into a comfortable position. To promote comfort, make sure you can breathe consistently and smoothly throughout.

√ Always extend as far as it feels comfortable, keeping in mind that everyone has a different range of comfort

3.2 Ankle to Knee

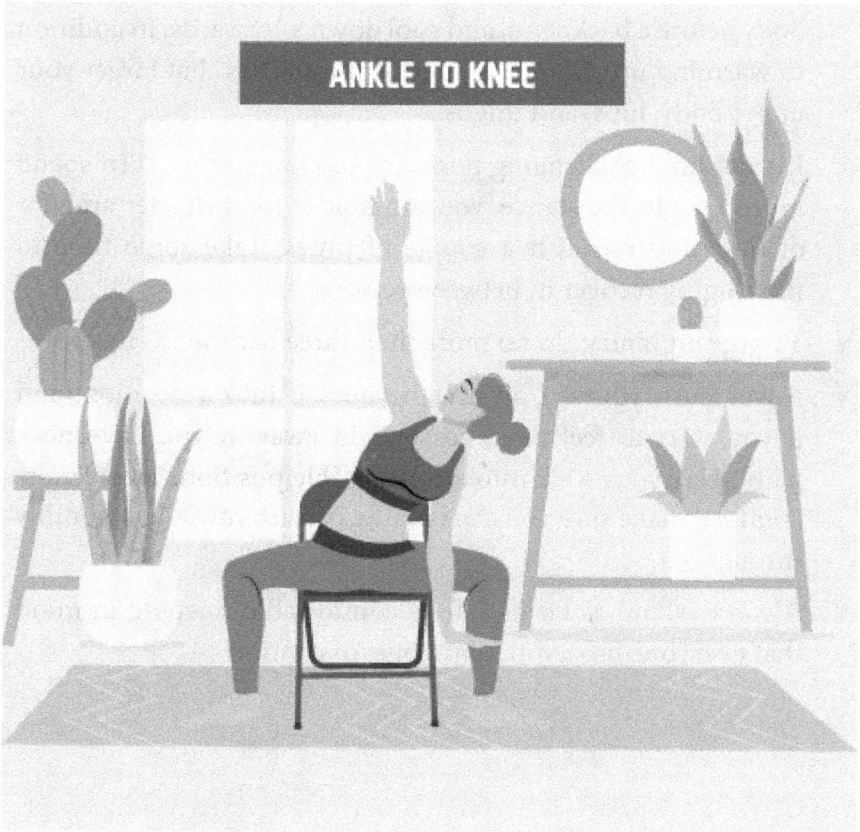

One of the main stress points in this exercise is the hip region. Follow these steps:

1. Sit up straight.

2. Bend your right knee.

3. Cross the right ankle above your left knee to ease the tension.

4. Lean forward to stretch more deeply.

5. After holding for five breaths, switch to the other side and repeat.

3.3 Reach Back

This workout stretches your chest and shoulders while enhancing your shoulder range of motion. It can feel comfortable to slouch when we stand or sit with our shoulders stooped forward. However, when we contract those muscles, our chests become tense. It may result in pain in our upper and mid-back if certain muscles are avoided. The exercise that follows, strengthens the postural muscles, opens up the chest, and enhances shoulder extension. Observe the directions provided:

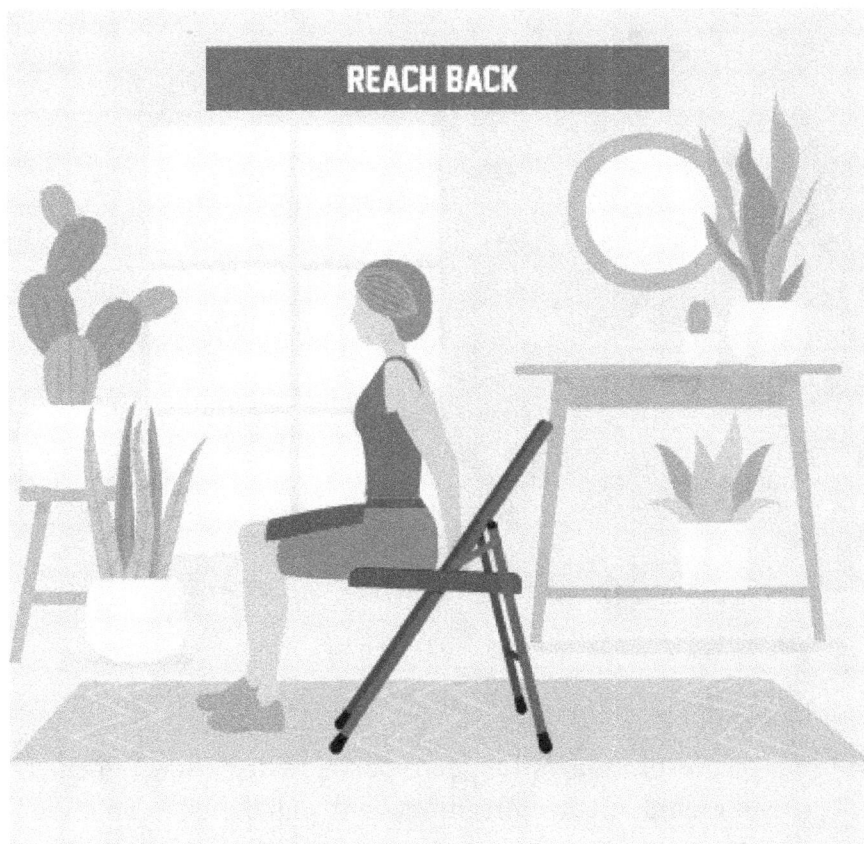

1. Sit firmly on the floor. Extend your spine.

2. Inhale deeply and stretch behind you and entangle your hands

as you exhale.

3. If you are unable to interweave your fingers, grab the opposing elbows or wrists.

4. Take a second deep breath and watch as you stand taller and your spine lengthens.

5. Roll your shoulders up and back while moving your shoulder

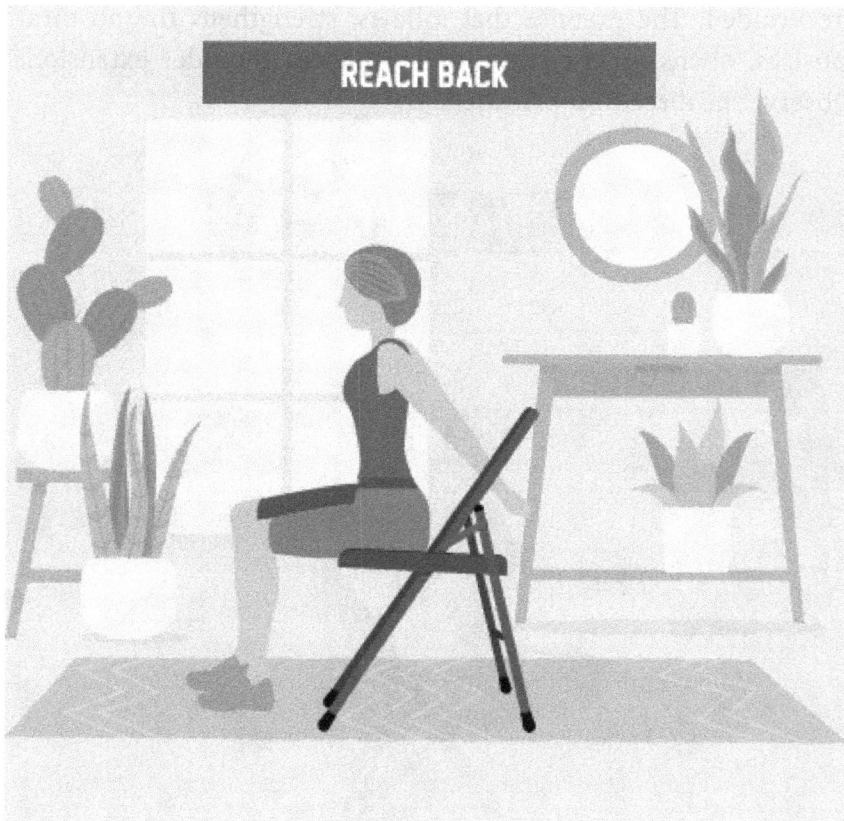

REACH BACK

blades down your back.

1. As you breathe, softly straighten your hands if they are clenched. (If your hands are not already clasped, pull lightly in opposing directions.) As a result, your upper back will bulge upward.

2. After three deep breaths, unclasp and return to neutral.

3. Repeat this process three more times.

3.4 Open Your Shoulders and Chest

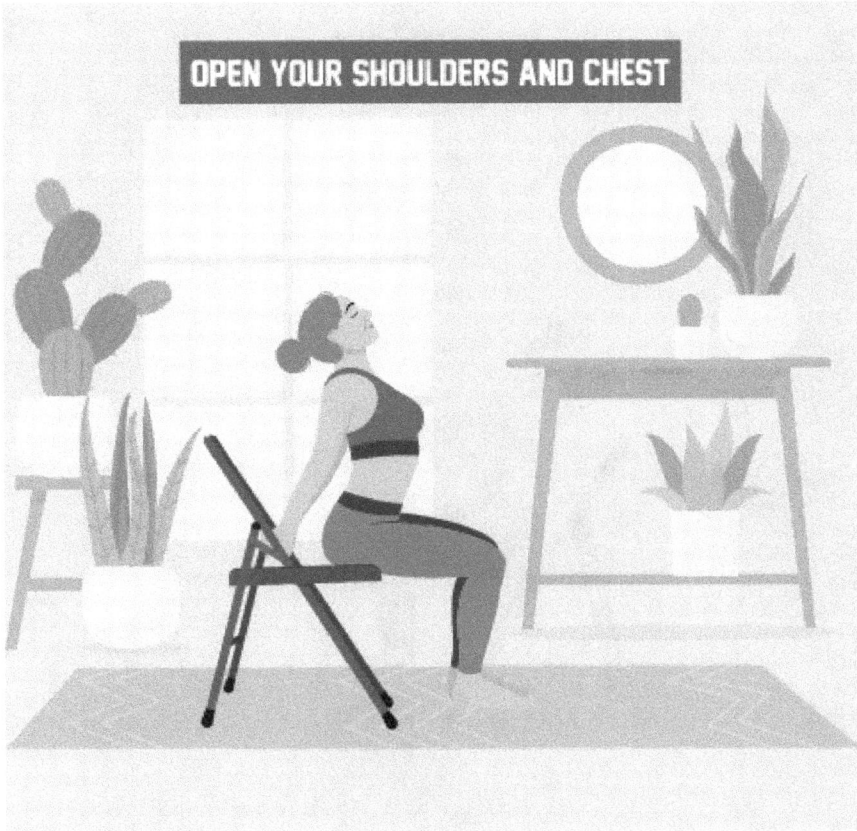

For this pose, follow these steps:

1. Bring your arms to your lower back and slowly draw your arms closer to each other until you encounter resistance. To do this, move yourself to the edge of your chair.

2. Stay in this position and take six calm, deep breaths, helping yourself relax in the pose as soon as you sense resistance.

3. Rolling out the shoulders will help you exit the stance as you slowly release your arms.

3.5 Mindful Mix

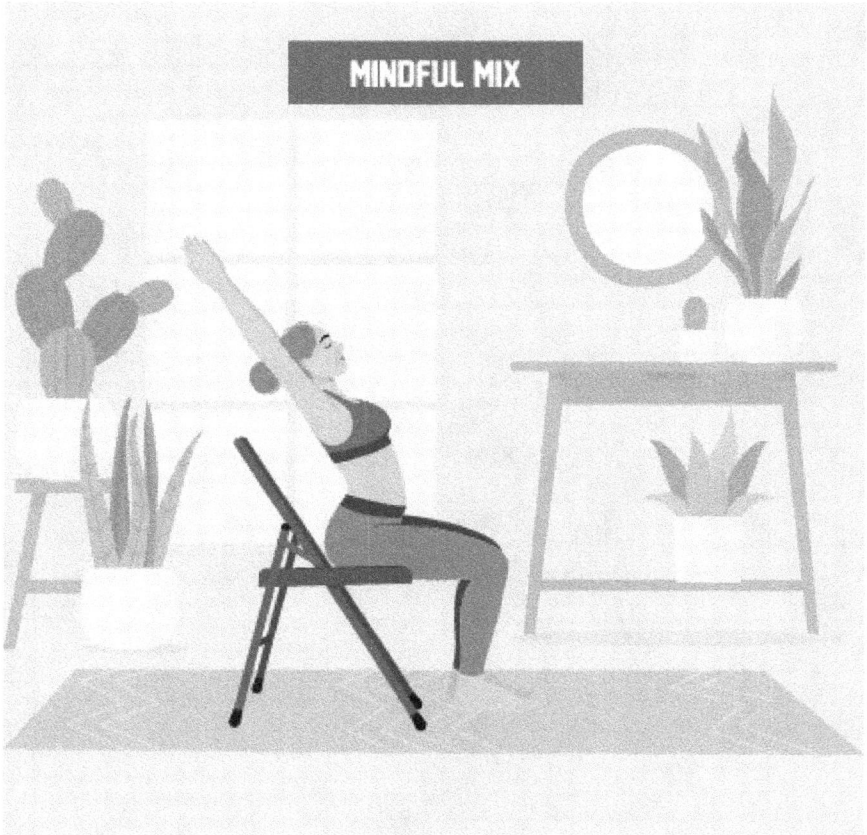

Place your head up toward the ceiling while keeping both of your feet firmly on the ground in the middle of the chair. Observe your body. Do you feel achy or tight in any area? What aspects of your body's experiences correspond to your day's tension or relaxation?

1. Gradually extend your breath. Feel your spine lengthen as you inhale, and your head's crown rises toward the ceiling. With each breath, gently tighten your abdominal muscles to straighten your lower back. With each inhale, let the abdominal muscles loosen up. This way, breathe for 5 to 10 breaths.

2. Move both arms overhead and to the sides, as you breathe in,

palms facing inward in direction of the ears. Move your arms back to the sides as you exhale, and softly tuck your chin into the hollow of the throat. Repeat 4–6 times.

3. Your palms should be facing inward when you hold the sides of the chair's back. Lean your ribcage ahead and move away from the chair while you softly press your shoulder blades together during an inhalation. There should be a slight backbend quality to this. Release back up to sitting and exhale. Repeat this motion six times, after which you should lean forward while taking four breaths, raising your ribs each time.

4. Bring the palms to the top of your thighs, starting from the seated position in posture 1. Extend your head upwards as you inhale. Move your hands towards the end of your legs and lean forward as you exhale. With each subsequent breath, lift your ribs with the aid of your hands and return to sitting by coming via a flattened position. Repeat 6–8 times.

5. From your starting seated pose in posture 1, raise your arms towards the side and upwards toward the sky while inhaling. Lace your fingers together. Press your palms upwards. Stretching the ribs, lean to the side while exhaling. Maintain a light belly contraction and make an effort to maintain shoulders that are parallel to one another. Move the torso back to the centre on an inhalation, and then exhale to the opposing side. Alternate sides and repeat this 4 times on each side.

6. Repetition of posture number 5, but this time fold forward on expiration and sweep both arms to the side and up to the ceiling on the inhalation. Stay folded forward for six breaths after completing 6 repetitions. Completely release all physical tension. Return to sitting after inhaling.

7. Return to posture number 1, which is a comfortable seated position with both feet firmly on the floor and the crown of your head raised toward the ceiling. Re-observe your body

this time with no bias. What effects did these exercises have on your body, breathing, emotions, and ability to concentrate?

3.6 Seated Pigeon Pose

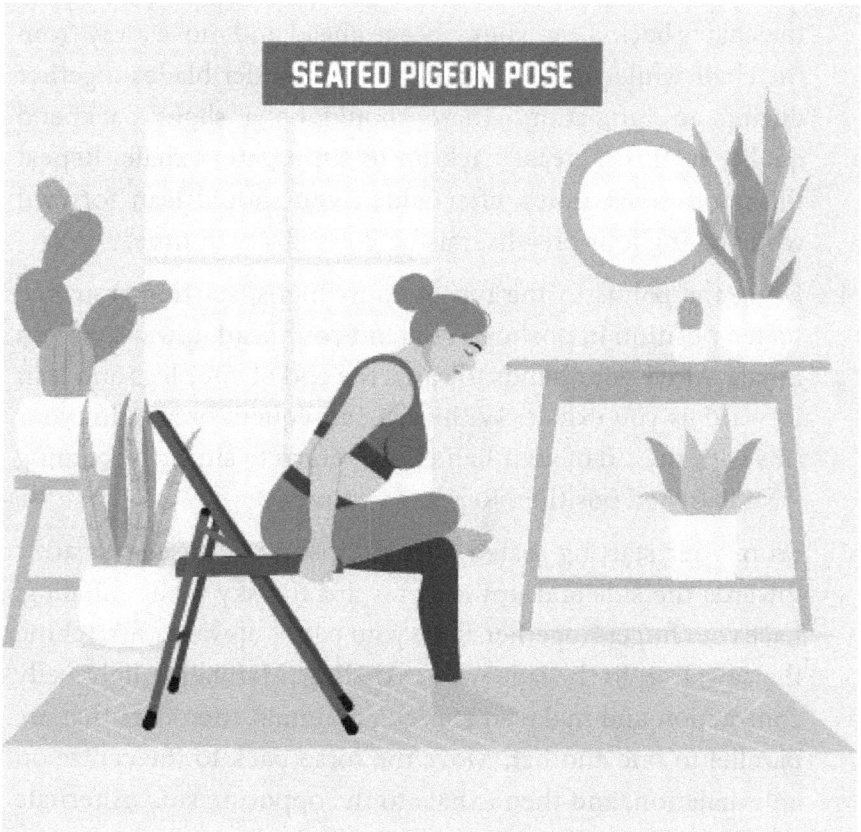

The seated pigeon posture, which is somewhat similar to crossing your legs is the best way to relax your hips. I have mentioned the steps below you need to follow:

1. While sitting still in a chair, open your right hip slightly to the side, elevate your right leg, and place your right ankle just over your left knee on your left thigh.

2. Continue to flex your right foot (it will activate the muscles around the right knee and protect it).

3. As the right knee bends toward the ground, feel the right hip release gradually while maintaining a straight spine.

Optional: You can gently press your right knee away from you by placing your right hand on your right thigh. Here, take up to ten breaths, then switch sides.

3.7 Seated Gomukhasana

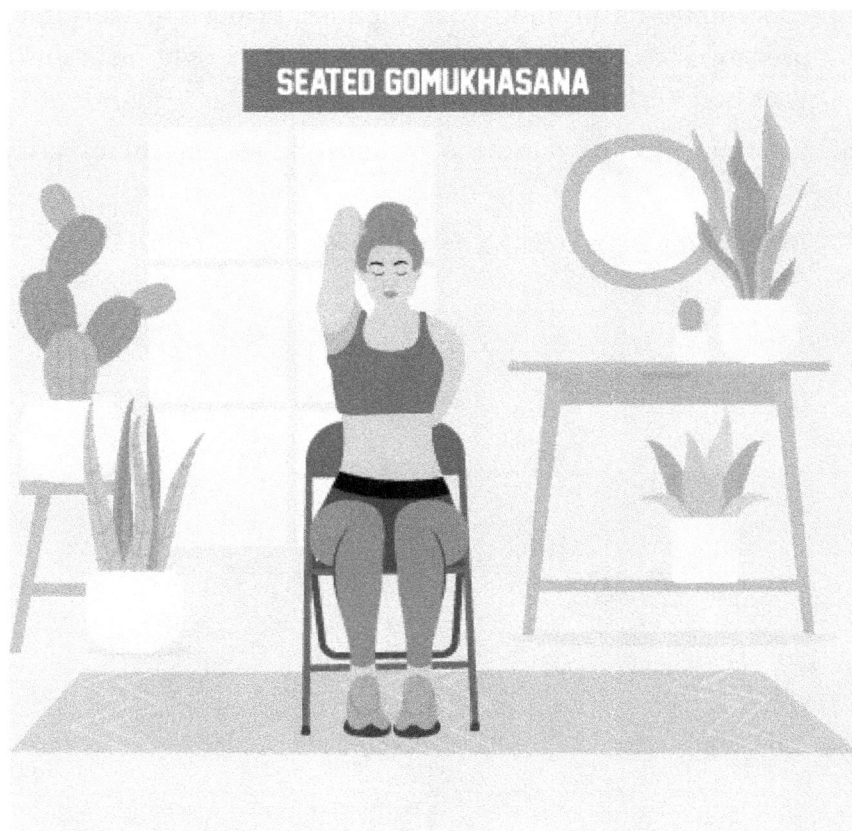

SEATED GOMUKHASANA

Gomukhasana is a wonderful pose for stretching your arms, opening your heart and shoulders, and straightening your upper back.

1. Place your right hand on the side of your chair and point your thumb downward. The right hand's back should be on your

back when you bend your elbow.

2. Put your left hand straight out in front of you with the palm facing up.

3. Bending the elbow, raise the left hand to the sky.

4. Your left palm should be on your back.

5. Instead of worrying about clasping your hands together, concentrate on pushing your shoulder blades together and pressing your left palm and the back of your right hand into your back (drawing the elbows back).

6. Continue pushing your heart forward and keeping an upward gaze.

7. After taking a few breaths, switch sides.

3.8 Back Circles

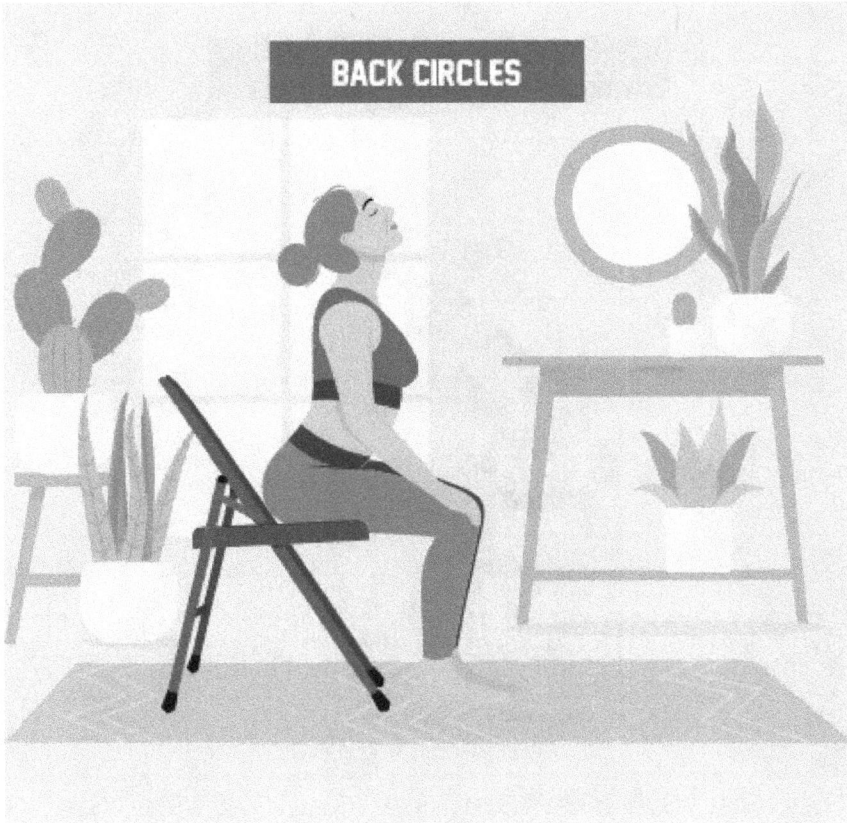

Here is how you can go about this posture exercise.

1. Remaining seated, rest the hands on knees for strong support and safety as you start to twist your torso in circular movements.

2. Step your feet slightly wider than they would naturally fall.

3. As your belly stays soft throughout your rotations, you will feel your chest expanding forward.

4. Try to pull your belly toward your spine in assisting your lower end of the back to bend.

5. I suggest doing this motion ten - twelve times in all directions to benefit from it the most.

3.9 Open up Side of Your Body

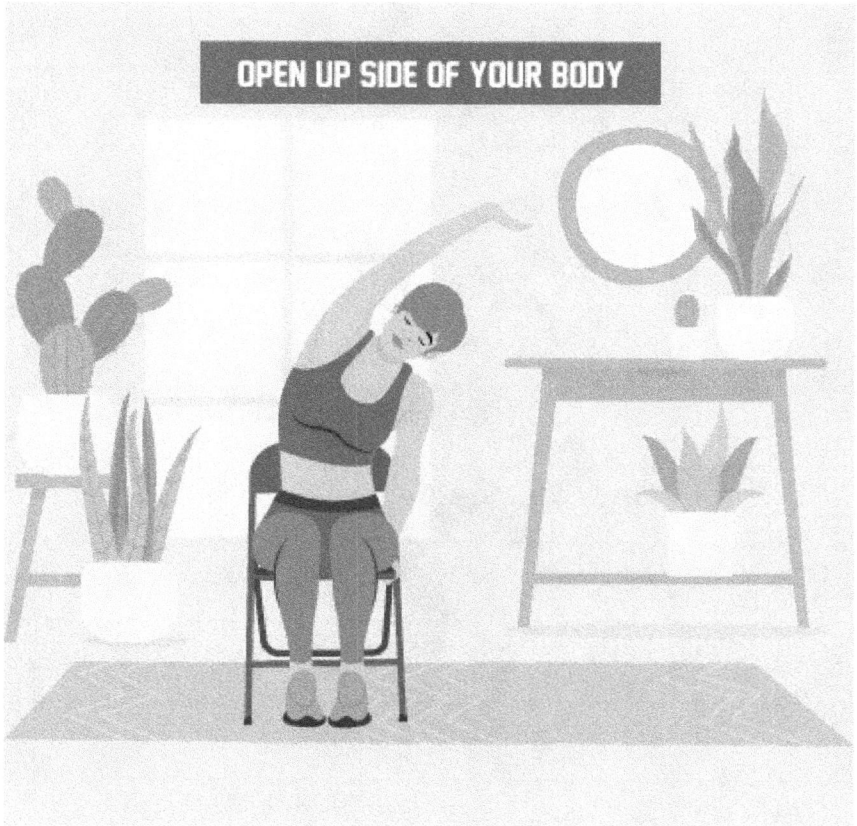

Below are the steps for this yoga pose.

1. Have a long stretch across the side of your body, sit up straight in your chair and raise your left arm.

2. Gently allow it to move towards the right side of the body.

3. Repeat on the other side after taking five to six deep breaths to ease yourself into the pose.

3.10 Neck Release

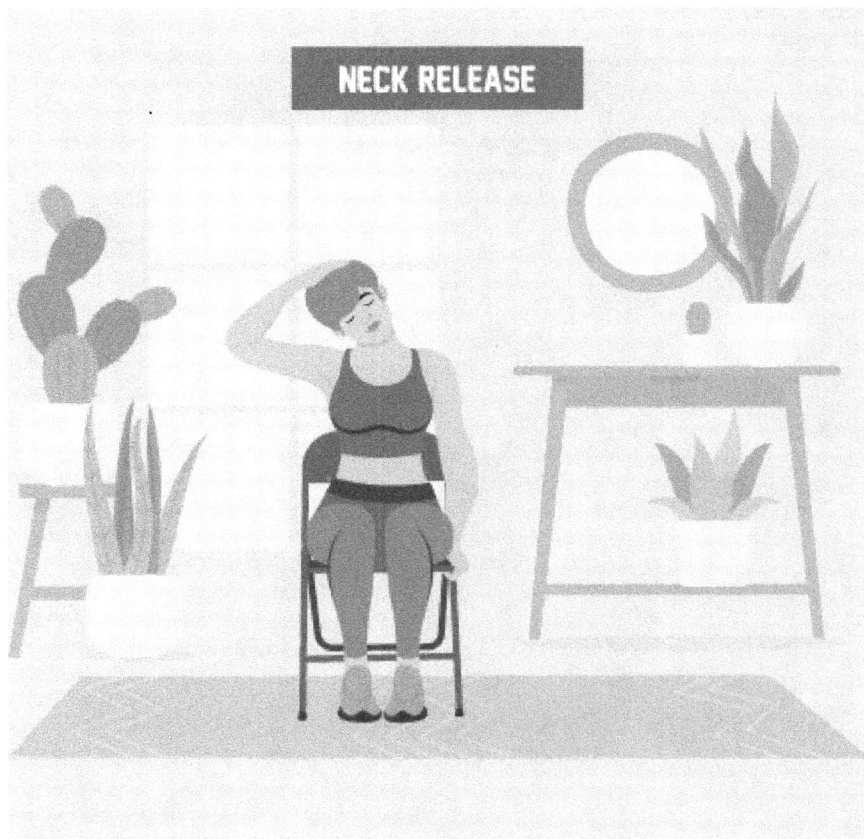

This yoga pose will help you loosen up your muscles.

1. Put your right hand above your left ear.

2. Allow your right ear to now droop toward your right shoulder.

3. Try to find a nice stretch from the left ear to the left shoulder in that stance, but go slowly.

4. You can experiment a little with your neck's angle, so lift and tuck your chin to get the best feelings.

5. Just let gravity work its magic; do not exert any pressure; the weight of your hand should be sufficient.

6. After taking a few breaths, switch sides.

3.11 Higher Alter Side Leans

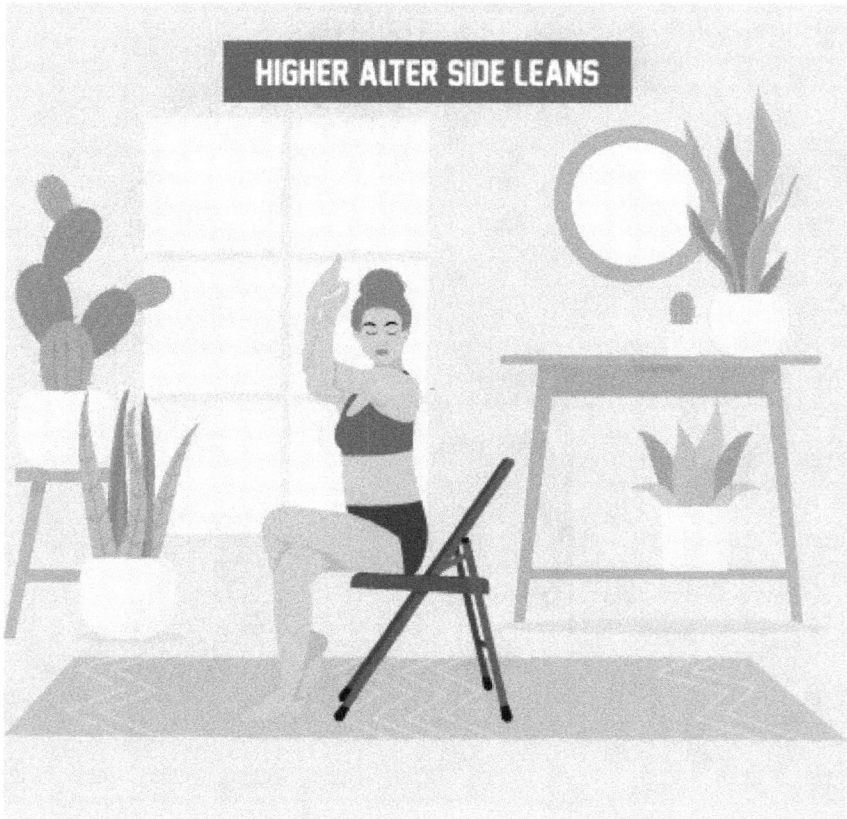

You need to follow these steps for higher alter side leans:

1. Raise your arms over your head and entwine your fingers in front of you for a powerful spine and shoulder stretch.

2. Next, straighten your arms above your head while turning your palms upward.

3. For three breaths, lean to the right, then for three to the left.

3.12 Sat Down Hip Opener

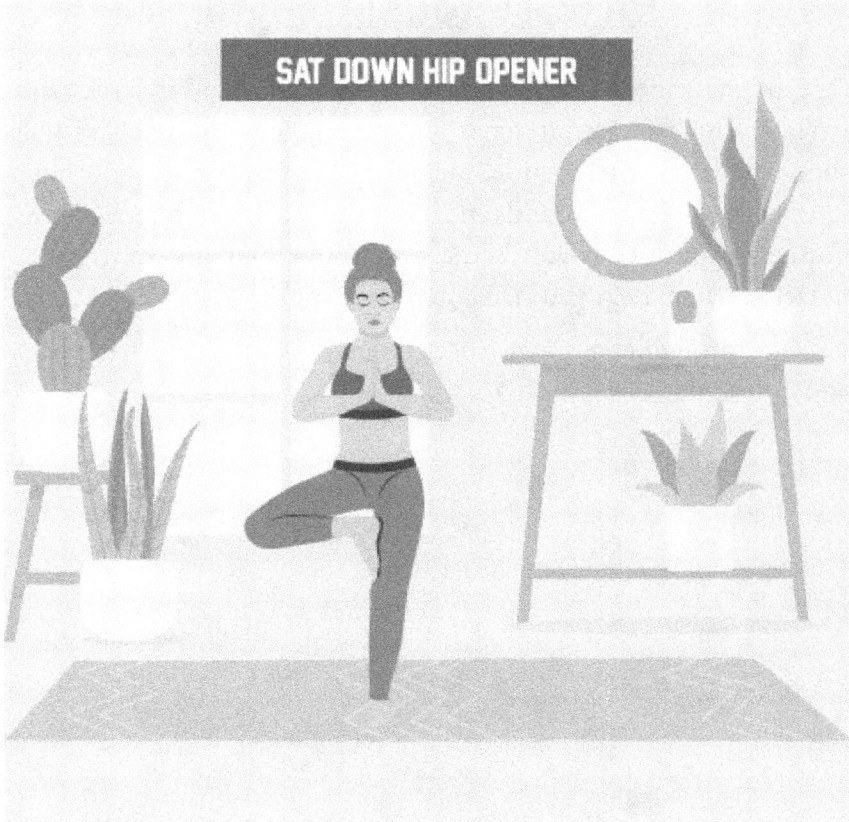

SAT DOWN HIP OPENER

For this pose, follow these steps:

1. Place your left ankle here and slowly raise it to the right knee.

2. Before putting your foot back on the floor and doing it again on the other side, take ten slow, deep breaths to relax into the motion.

3. Stay in the pose for as long as you want if you notice that you are tenser in this area.

These yoga poses will help you minimize your muscle and joint strain by working on your posture.

Chapter 4: Get Rid of Back Pain and Increase Your Strength

One of the more effective methods for easing lower back pain is yoga. The exercise stretches and strengthens the muscles that support the back and spine, including the transverse abdominis in the belly, which also aids in spinal stabilization, the multifidus muscles, which help you bend your spine, and the Para spinal muscles, which help you straighten your spine.

Let's go through chair yoga poses that will relieve your back pain and boost your body strength.

4.1 Chair Cat-Cow

This well-known position lengthens the spine both forward and backwards. It works wonders for those who have bad posture. It is frequently carried out at the start of a yoga exercise to assist the muscles along the spine in warming up. Here are the steps you need to follow:

1. Start by placing your hands on your knees and your feet on the ground.

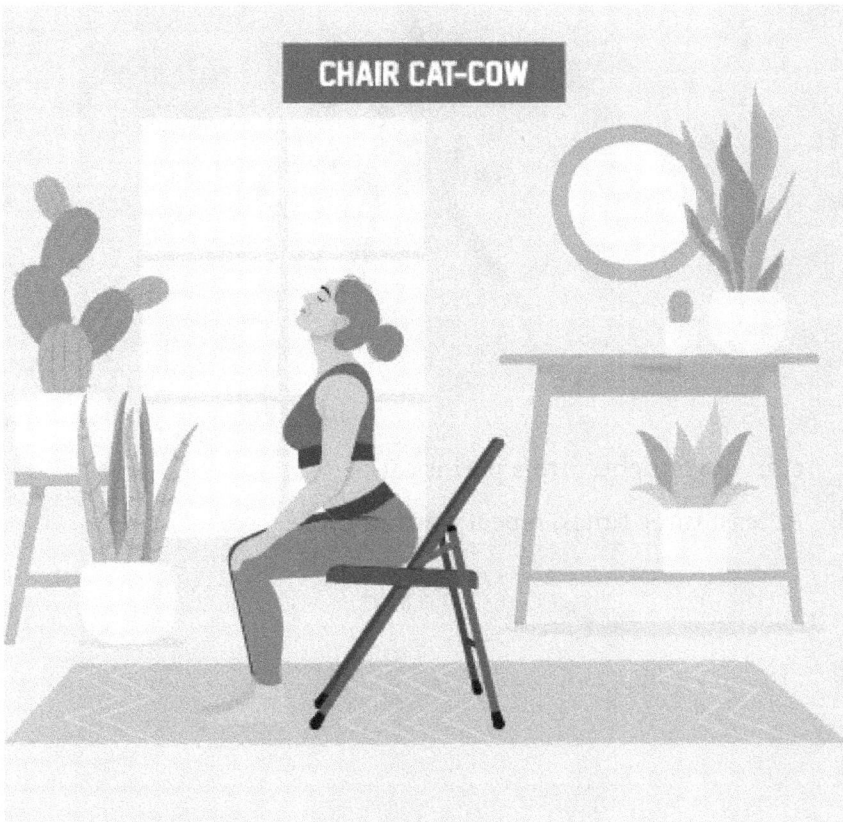

2. Inhale and extend your chest (this part is cow).

3. Stretch your spine the other way as you exhale, bringing your

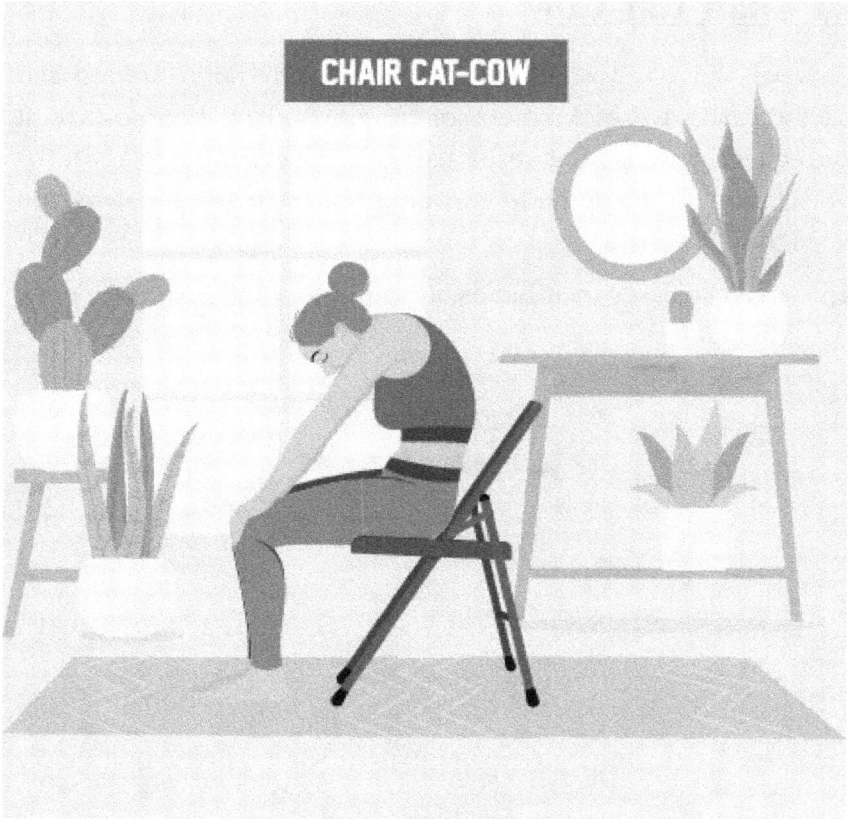

chin to your chest (this part is cat).

4. At least three times, repeat this full cycle.

4.2 Chair Upward Salute

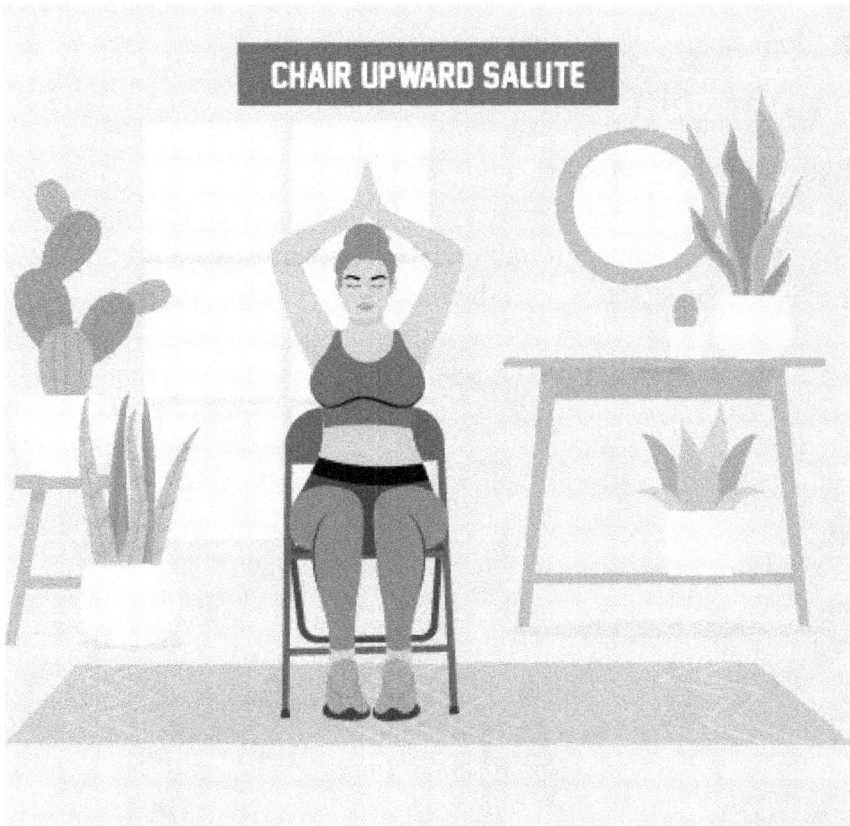

In addition to strengthening the core, this pose extends and strengthens the sides of the body.

1. Put your hands together and sit up straight to begin.

2. As you relax your shoulders and back and engage your buttocks and core, raise your palms toward the ceiling.

3. Exhale and keep reaching up as you begin to arch to the right.

4. As you lean to the right, another variant is to grip your left wrist with your right hand.

5. For two to five breaths, maintain the position.

6. Inhale and move back to the center in order to exit the right-facing arch.

7. Repeat on your left after that.

4.3 Warrior I

Extending the hip flexors, ankle, calf muscle, foot, and quadriceps, this position will relieve tension. The soreness in the low back, which is frequently brought on by tight muscles straining the pelvis, can be lessened with the release of this tension.

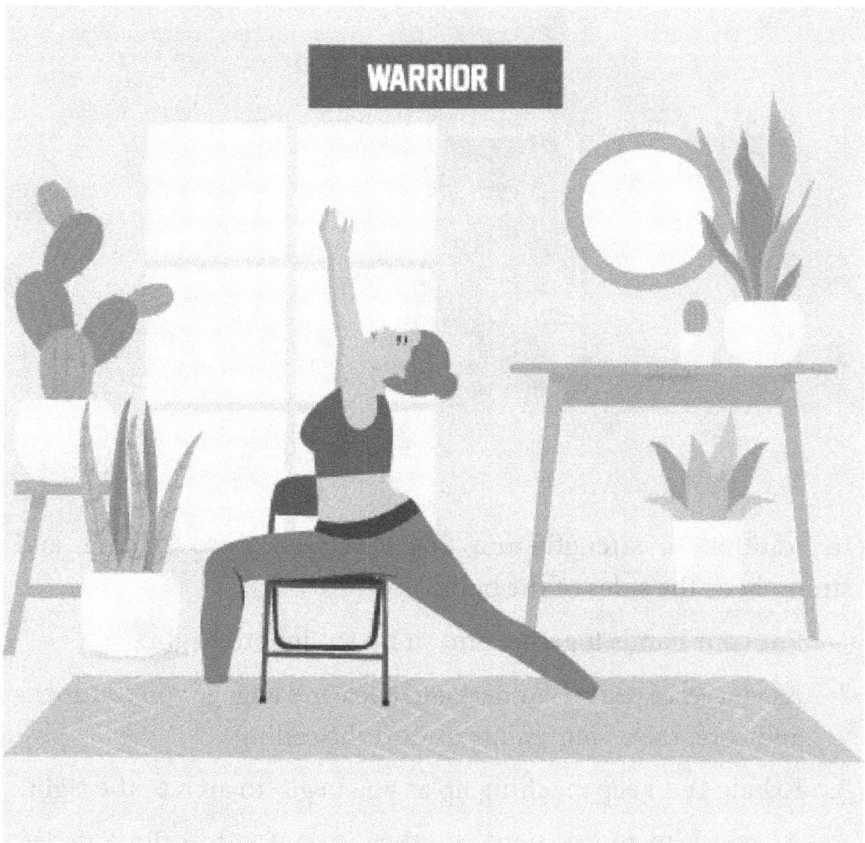

WARRIOR I

Here is how you can do the warrior I pose:

1. Your left leg should be placed off to the side of the chair as you

turn to the left while sliding to the edge of the chair.

2. Your back right leg should be extended behind you, with the foot as level as possible and the toes pointing slightly in the direction of the right corner of the room.

3. Move your hips slowly toward your left leg and lift your arms in front of you at shoulder height or higher, palms facing each other.

4. Imagine holding an apple between your shoulder blades to keep your shoulders relaxed.

5. If raising your arms hurts, consider lowering them a little.

6. If you enjoy a challenge, stomp your left foot's heel into the ground to engage your left quadriceps.

7. Repeat on the other side.

4.4 Thread the Needle

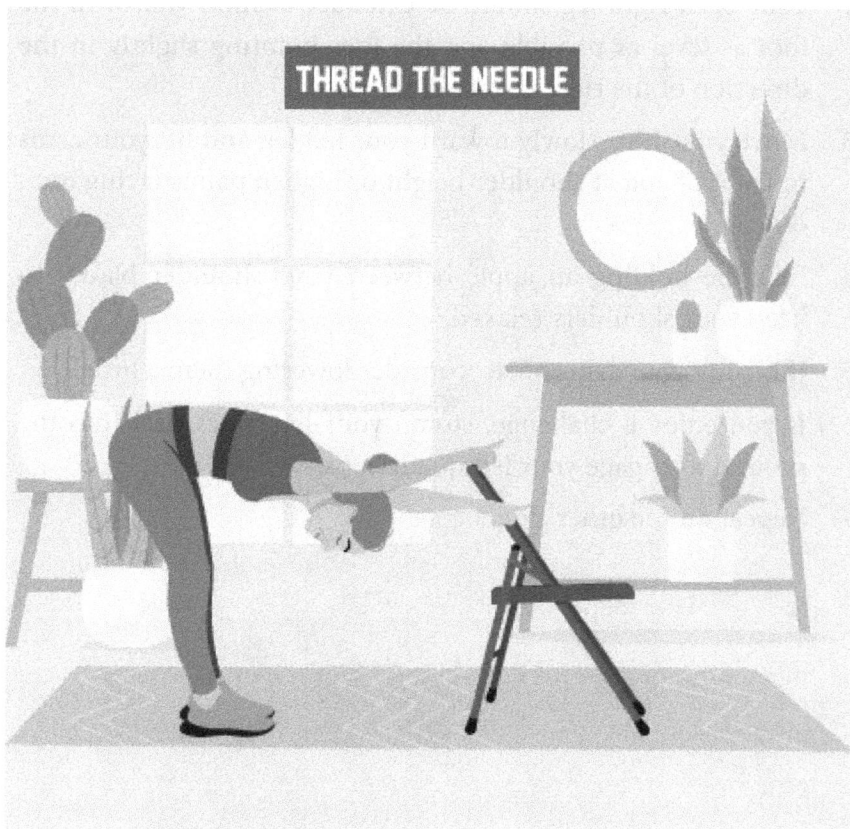

This little spine twist helps in easing the low back, neck, and shoulder strain. Regularly performing this pose can help relieve persistent back and shoulder pain. Here are the steps you need to follow:

1. Put your hands on the chair's back at about shoulder width while standing behind it.

2. Put your hands on the outside of the chair and take a step back with your feet as if performing a down dog.

3. Take a step ahead with the right leg.

4. You should feel relief on the right side of your torso when you

shift your weight back.

5. As you gently pull on the right hand, maintain your back flat and your abdominal muscles firm.

6. Repeat on the other side after holding the pose.

4.5 Lengthen the Spine

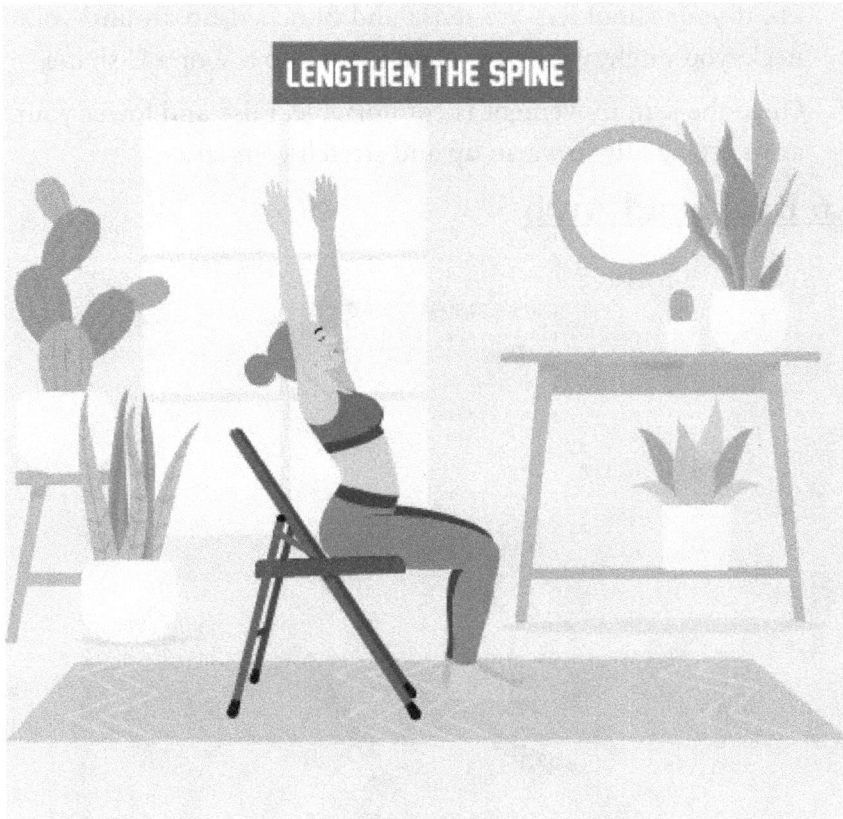

Below are some steps you must follow for this exercise:

1. Create more space between the vertebrae.

2. The spine's natural curvature should considerably be flattened and straightened in this posture.

3. Warm the shoulders as well.

4. Your feet should be flat on the floor beneath your knees, and you should sit on the very edge of your chair with your back straight.

5. Sweep your arms forward and upward, starting from your side, aiming for the ceiling.

6. Find a position where you are comfortable, and your arms are up; if your shoulders are tense and bunched up around your neck, you might want to expand them into a V or a U shape.

7. Once the arm movement is comfortable, raise and lower your arms repeatedly to warm up and stretch your spine.

4.6 Backbend Arch

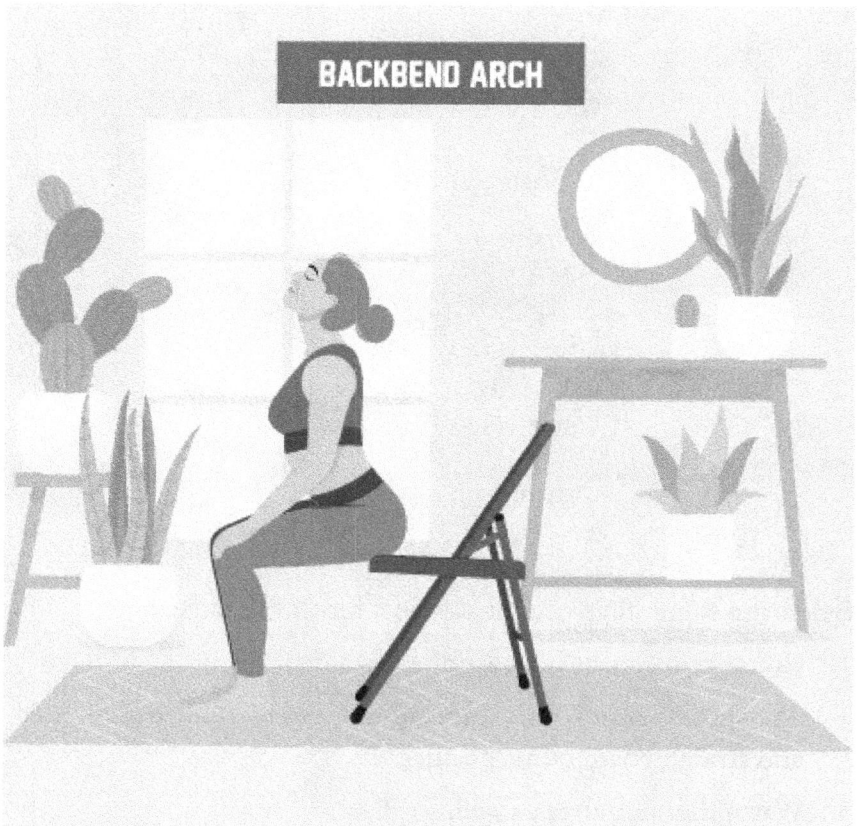

BACKBEND ARCH

Here is how you can go about backbend arch:

1. Starting at the edge of the chair, place your hands behind you with your fingers pointing away from your hips.

2. Using your fingertips as support, raise your lower back by pulling your sacrum in and upward.

3. Open out the entire front body by continuing the backbend all the way up to the shoulder blades.

4. For 8 to 10 breaths, hold the position, then let go.

4.7 Chair Single-leg Stretch

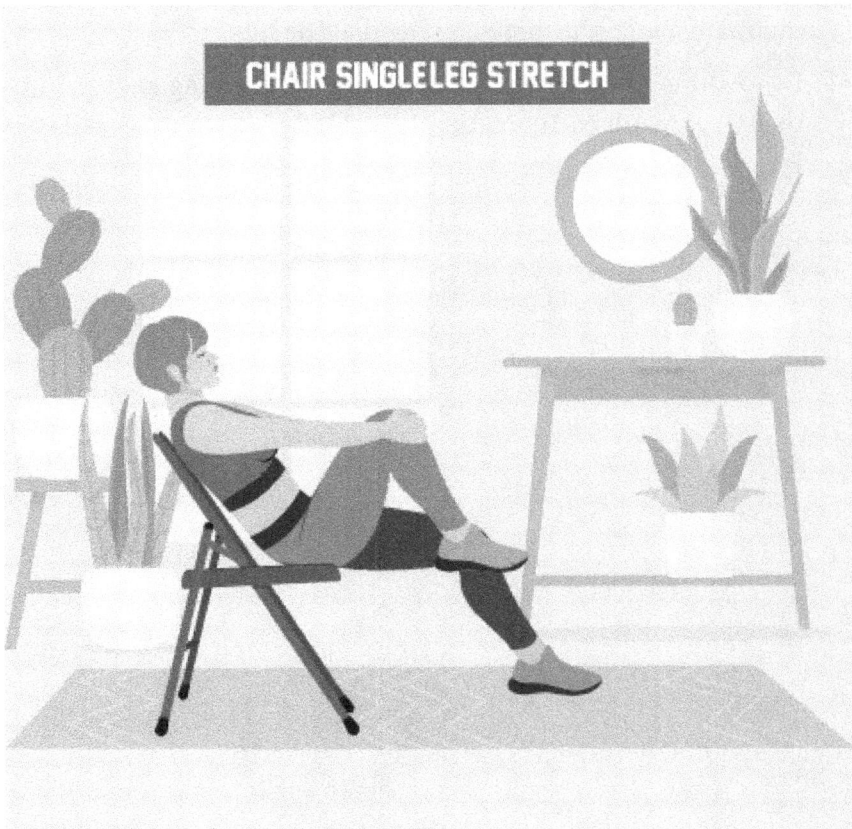

You will stretch your calves and hamstrings in this position. Here we go:

1. Sit close to the edge of your seat to start, but not too close so that you feel like you could fall off.

2. Straighten your right leg out and point your right toes upward while sitting upright.

3. Put your left foot flat on the ground and bend your left knee at a 45-degree angle.

4. As you exhale, carefully move your hands down your leg while keeping your spine straight and placing both hands on your leg.

5. The urge to lower your head to your leg must be resisted as you maintain a straight spine and bend at the hips.

6. Follow this for five breaths, progressively slipping deeper into the stretch with each breath.

7. Inhale as you slowly rise out of the posture, then switch sides.

4.8 Twist Left and Right

Here is how you can do the twist yoga pose.

1. Select a chair without arms and a flat seat.

2. Your feet should be flat on the floor beneath your knees, and you should sit on the very edge of your chair with your back straight.

3. Raise your arms to at most shoulder height, sway to one side, and then lower one arm to your knee and the other to the seat of the chair.

4. Return to the center and raise your arms once again.

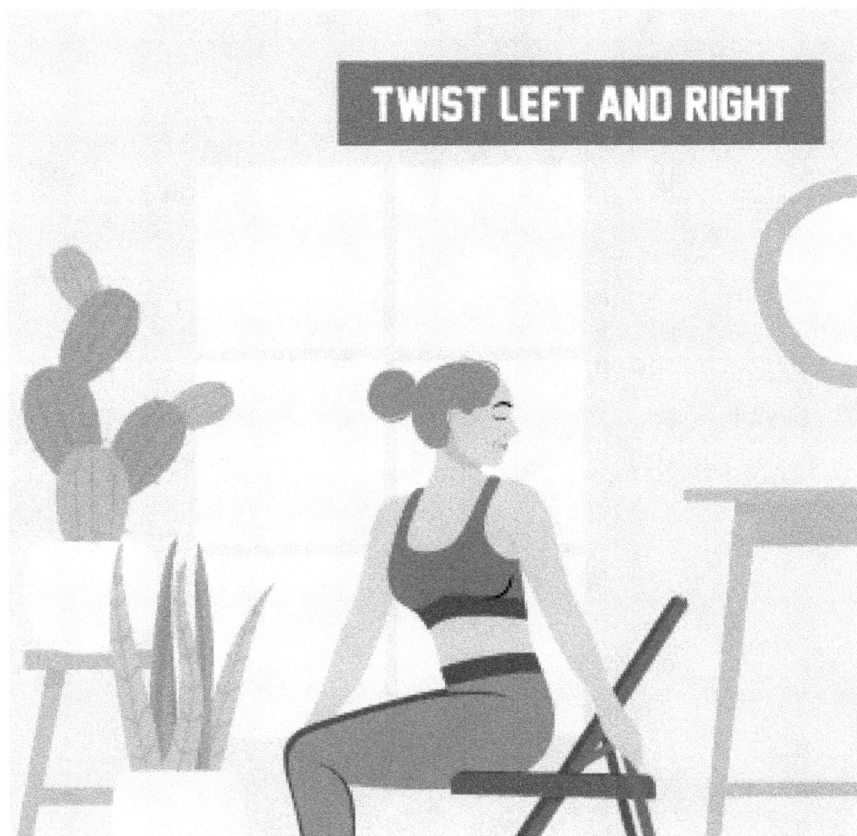

TWIST LEFT AND RIGHT

5. Put your arms down.

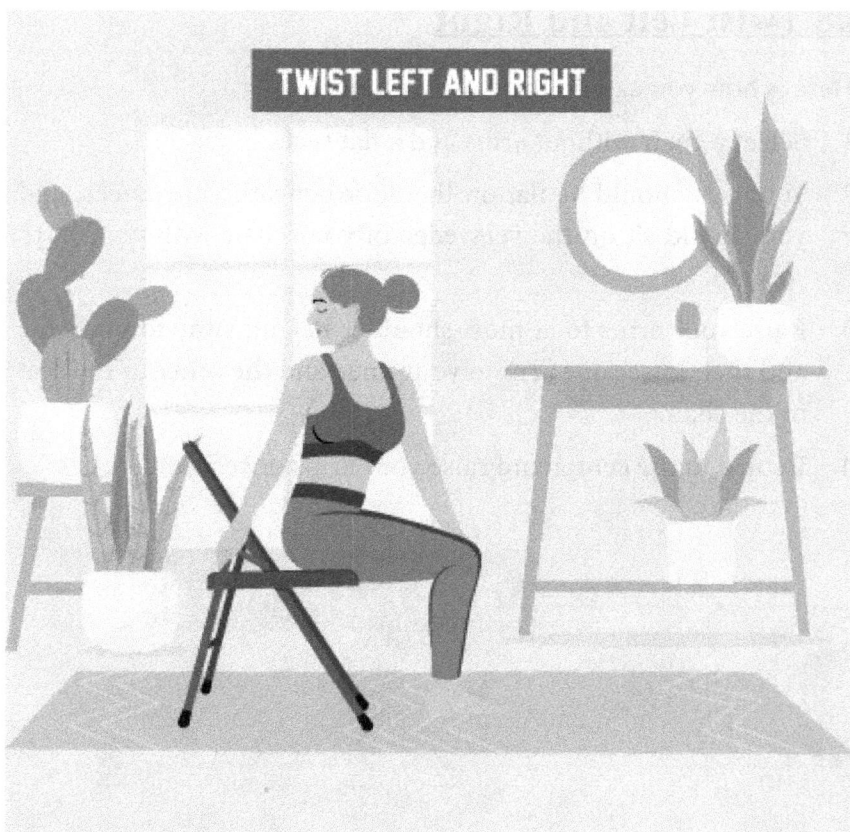

TWIST LEFT AND RIGHT

1. Repeat on the opposite side.

2. Do a few sets.

3. Always bend forward to counteract any negative effects.

4.9 Lower Back Circles

Here are the steps you need to follow:

1. Sit with feet hip-width apart and knees bent.

2. After taking a breath, start rotating your torso clockwise,

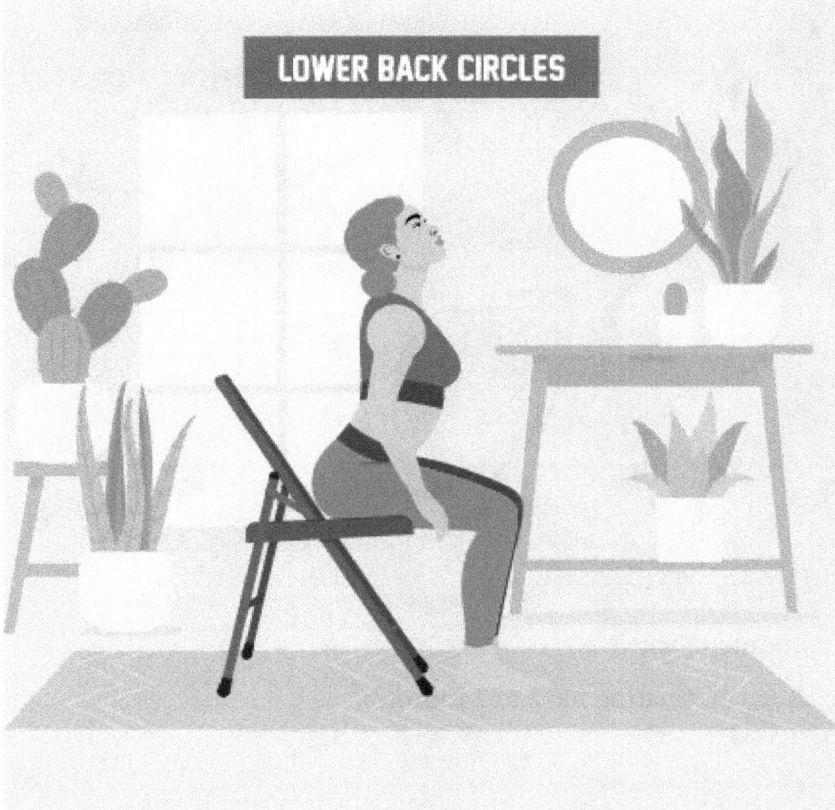

making careful to start at the base of your spine.

3. Finish eight to ten rotations.

4. Stop, and then carry out the motion once more while rotating

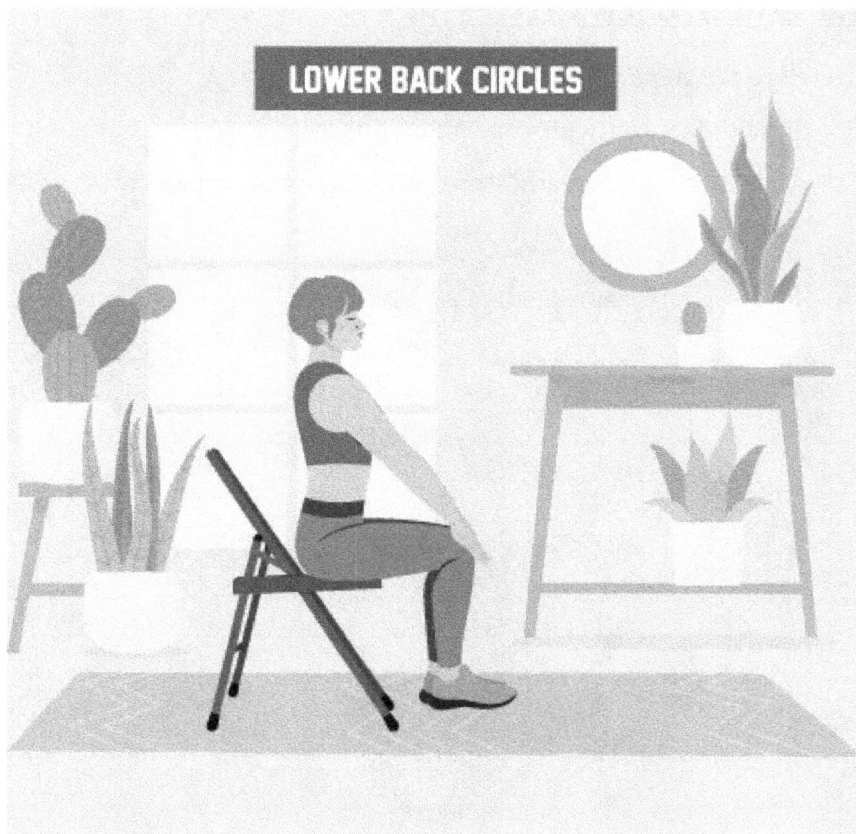

counterclockwise.

5. Keep alternating for 2 to 3 minutes.

4.10 Roll-Downs

Here is how you can do the roll-down pose:

1. Sit with your feet hip distance apart and your hands by your sides.

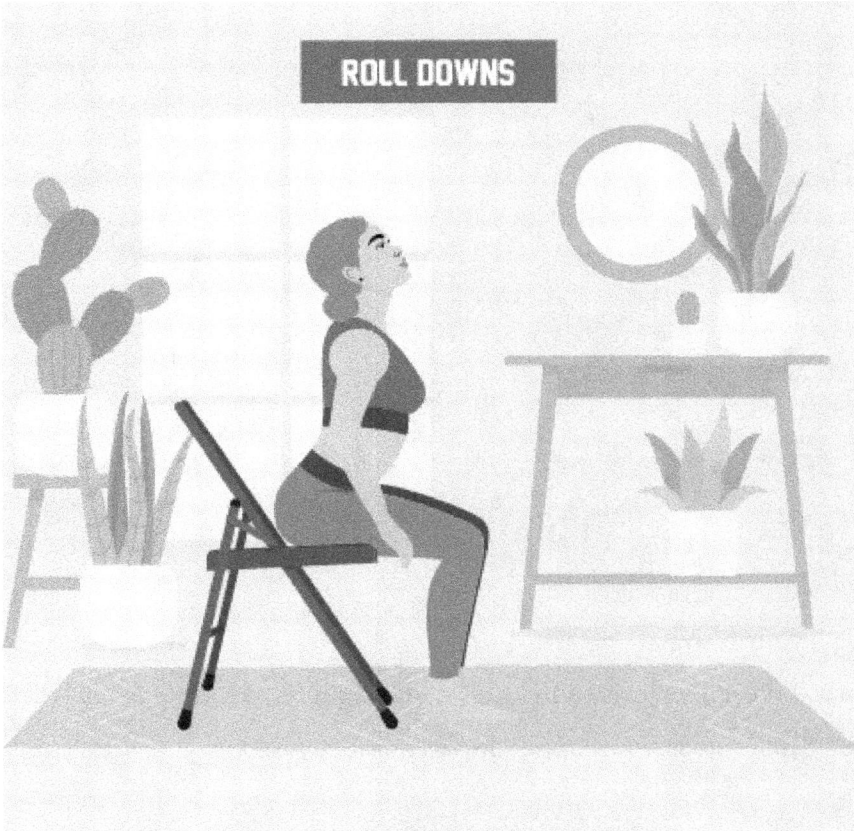

2. Beginning with the head, bend down through the spine.

3. Exhale, letting your forehead drop forward and allowing your head's weight to carry you over till your thighs are in front of

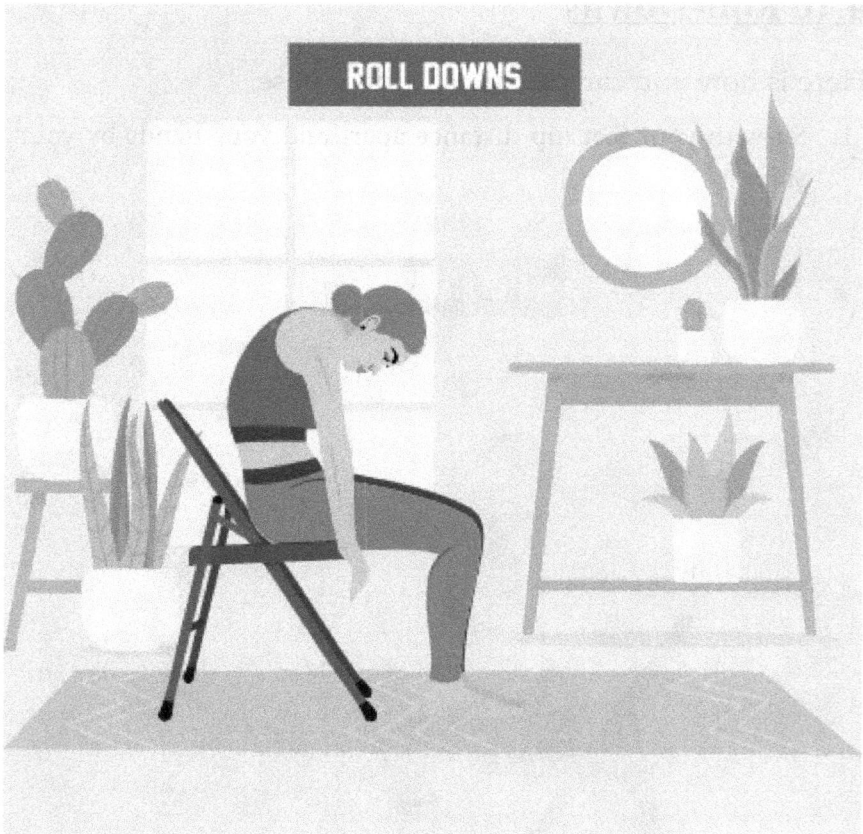

your brow.

4. Take a deep breath in and slowly begin to round up to sit.

5. To protect your back, draw your belly button close to your

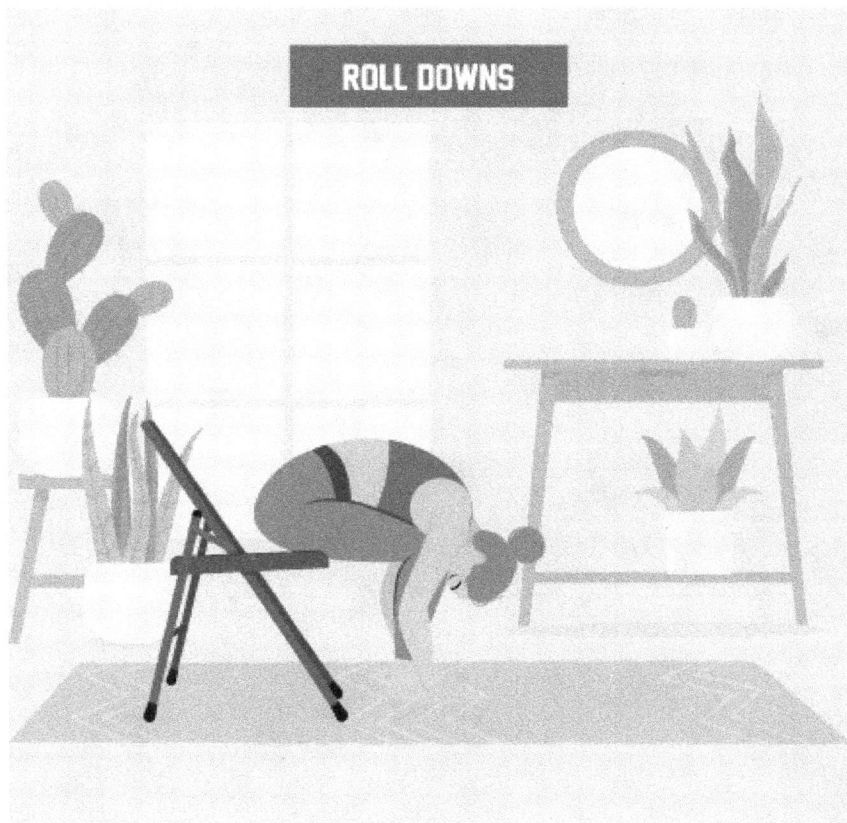

spine.

6. As you circle up, feel the articulation.

7. For five to eight cycles, keep rolling down and up.

4.11 Side Angle

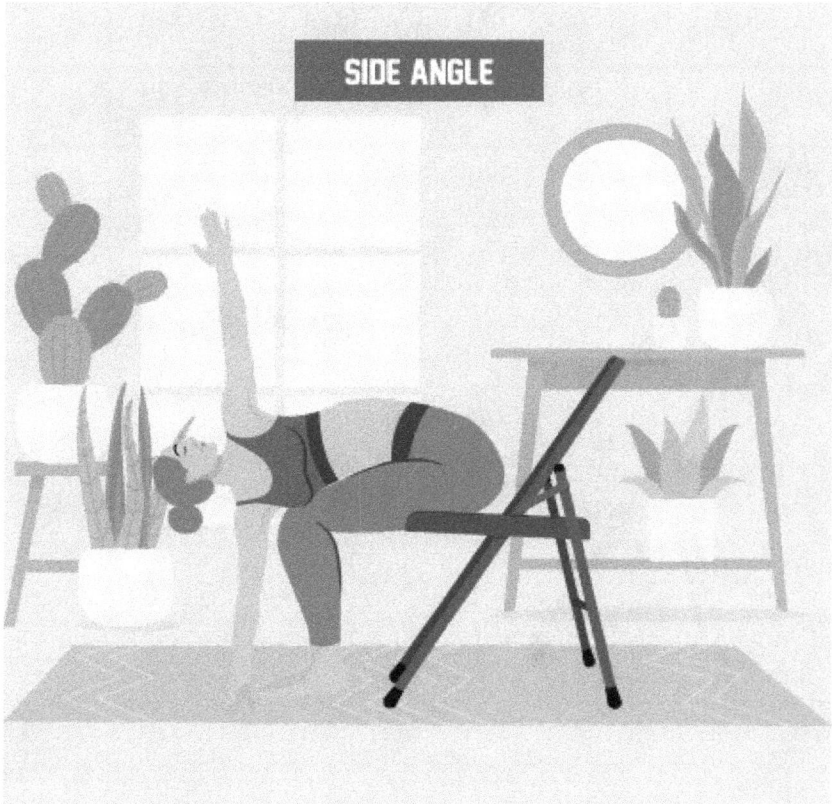

Your spine will be more flexible after doing this posture. Here is how you can do it:

1. While seated in a chair without wheels, stoop over and place your right palm outside of your left foot on the floor.

2. Raise your left arm toward the sky.

3. Turn your head to look at your left hand and arm.

4. Stretch for a second, then repeat on the other side.

5. Outside of your right foot, place your left palm on the ground.

6. Your right arm should be raised, and your eyes should be directed onto the right hand.

4.12 Lunge

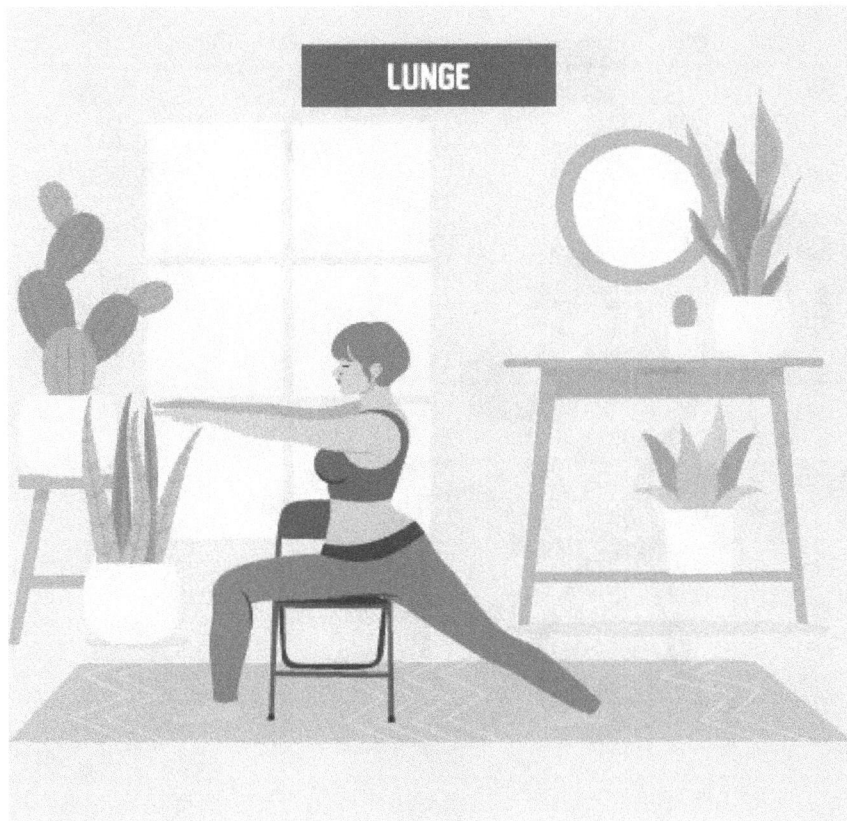

The lunge enables the relaxation of tension in the calf, ankle, foot, lower back, and hip flexors. The lunge is a suitable substitute for those who lack pelvic flexibility or find Warrior I difficult. While targeting the muscles at various angles to allow for a better release of tension across the area, this gives you very similar advantages as Warrior I. Here we go:

1. Hold the Warrior I position, turn your back foot, so the toes face forward, and press back with your raised heel.

2. Press the front heel firmly on the floor to add a quadriceps-strengthening element to the exercise.

4.13 Cobra Chair Pose

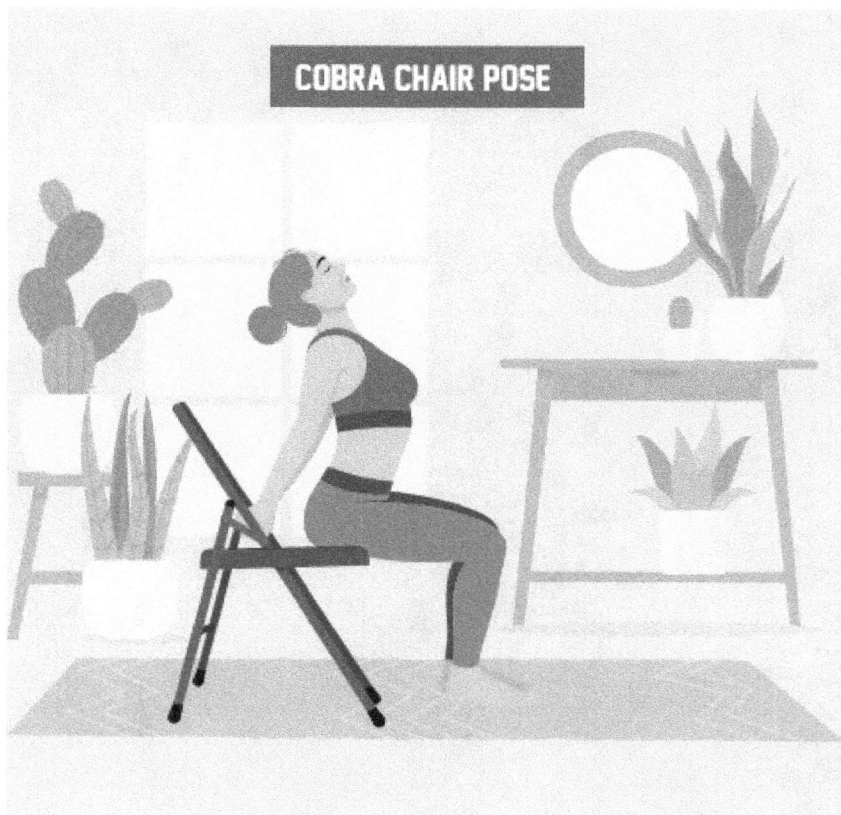

A backbend for beginners is called the cobra chair posture.

Your back, shoulders, chest, and hips can all be strengthened while releasing the tension, tightness, and pain with backbends. Because it lengthens your spine, develops flexibility, and enhances mobility, it also encourages proper posture. Here are the steps you need:

1. Hold a chair's back with your arms while sitting at the edge of your chair.

2. Lift your shoulders and chest to look up as you inhale.

3. You will feel a stretch in your upper chest and neck as you exhale.

4.14 Torso Flow

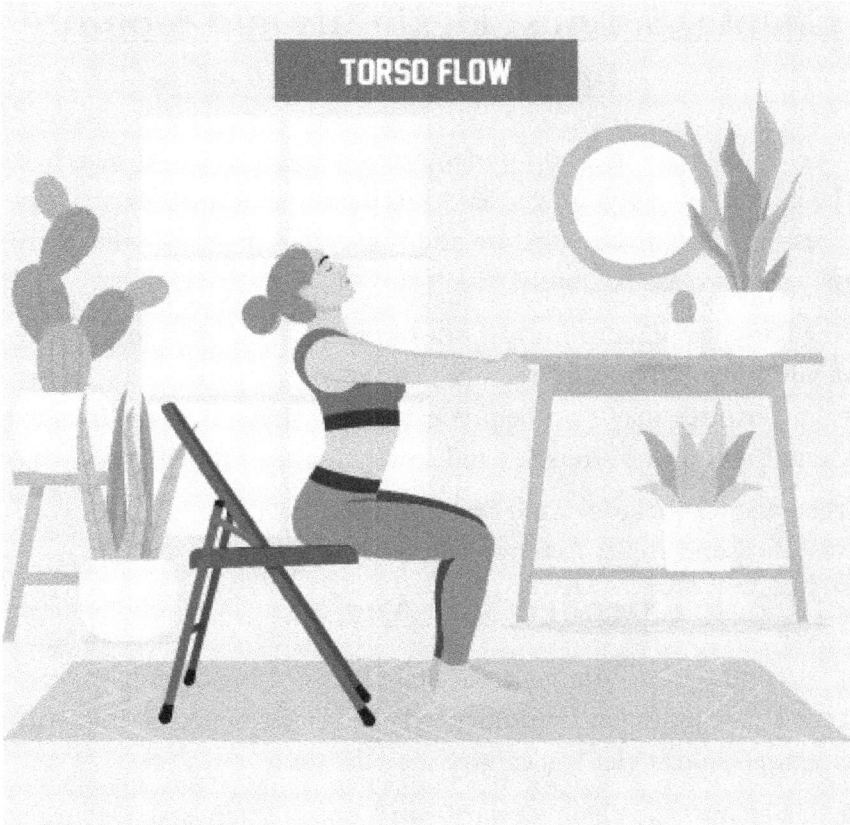

1. Interlace your fingers.

2. Inhale, palms facing away from your body.

3. Put your arms out straight.

4. Stretch your torso forward while pressing your palms forward.

5. Put your hands in the air and lift your torso high.

6. Exhale and move your arms to the side.

7. Repeat three to five times.

These yoga poses will help reduce back pain and strengthen your body. Let's move onto the next chapter.

Chapter 5: Boost Flexibility and Mobility for Your Wellbeing

One of the essential components of excellent physical health is flexibility. But as you age, lead a sedentary lifestyle, experience stress, or develop bad posture and movement patterns, your body may start to lose flexibility.

Regular yoga practice may be one of the best strategies to improve flexibility and increase mobility in your muscles and joints. Many yoga postures may also help you feel less stressed or anxious by strengthening your muscles and enhancing your flexibility.

This chapter includes chair yoga poses to help you get back your flexibility and ability to move around and walk.

5.1 Chair Extended Side Angle

This technique is similar to a chair forward bend with a twist. Your chest, lungs, and shoulders will be strengthened by the chair extended side angle. You can try it by the following steps:

1. Fold into the chair-forward-bend pose (Uttanasana). Place a yoga block on the outside of the left foot or the floor with the left fingertips.

2. As you breathe in, open your chest and turn to the right. Your right arm should be raised toward the ceiling while you inspect it.

3. Repeat on the other side after holding for a while.

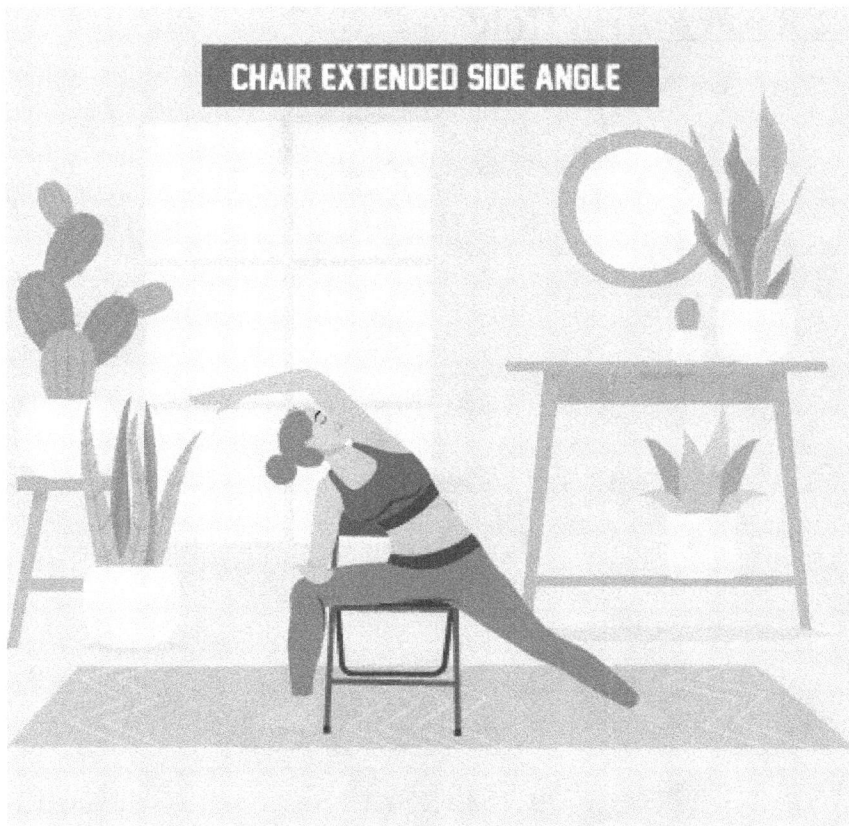

CHAIR EXTENDED SIDE ANGLE

You can modify it easily if you cannot touch the floor with ease. You can use a block or some other substantial item.

5.2 Reverse Arm Hold

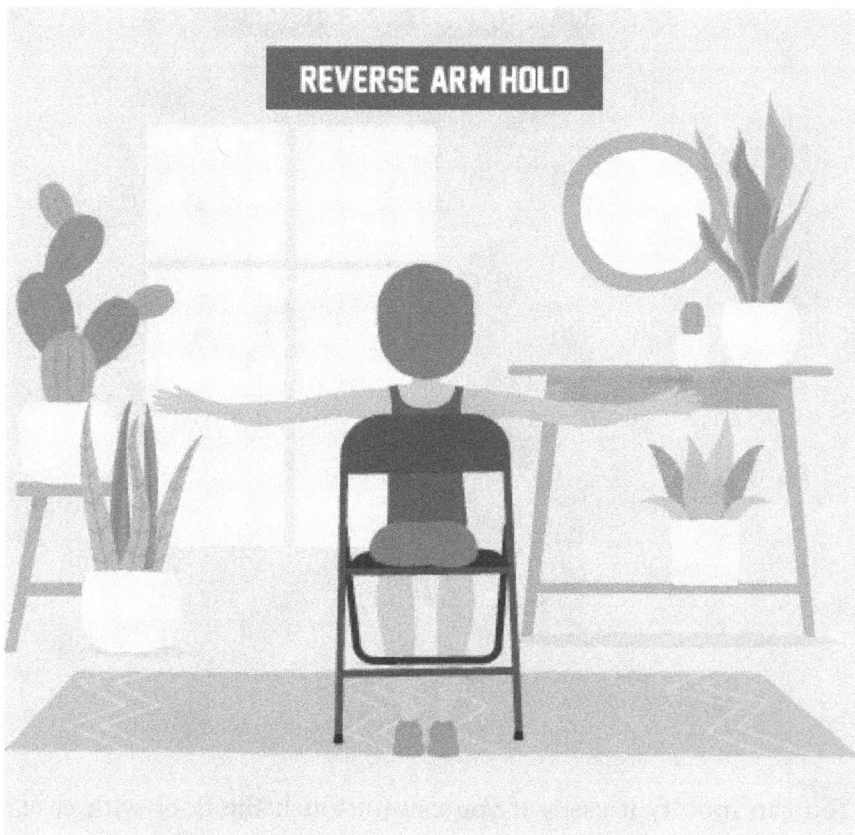

The Reverse Arm Hold elongates your arms, widens your chest, and promotes relaxation.

1. Inhale as you extend your arms on the sides, palms facing down. As you exhale, move both shoulders forward. Let your hands swing loosely behind your back.

2. To add some resistance, clasp your hands together and pull softly. Do not let go of your hold, though.

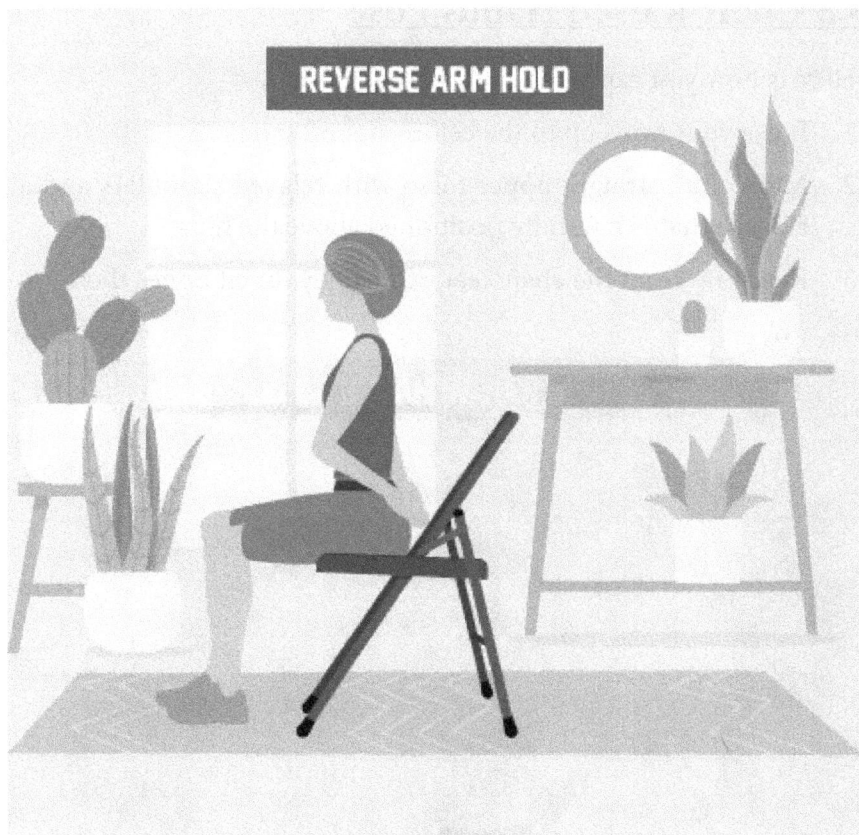

REVERSE ARM HOLD

3. Repeat with the opposite arms after five long breaths.

5.3 Chair Raised Hands Pose

Here is how you can go about this yoga pose:

1. Raise your arms up to the ceiling as you inhale.

2. Maintain a straight upper torso with relaxed shoulders and a ribcage that is naturally positioned above the hips.

3. Reach up from the chair seat, securing your sit bones there.

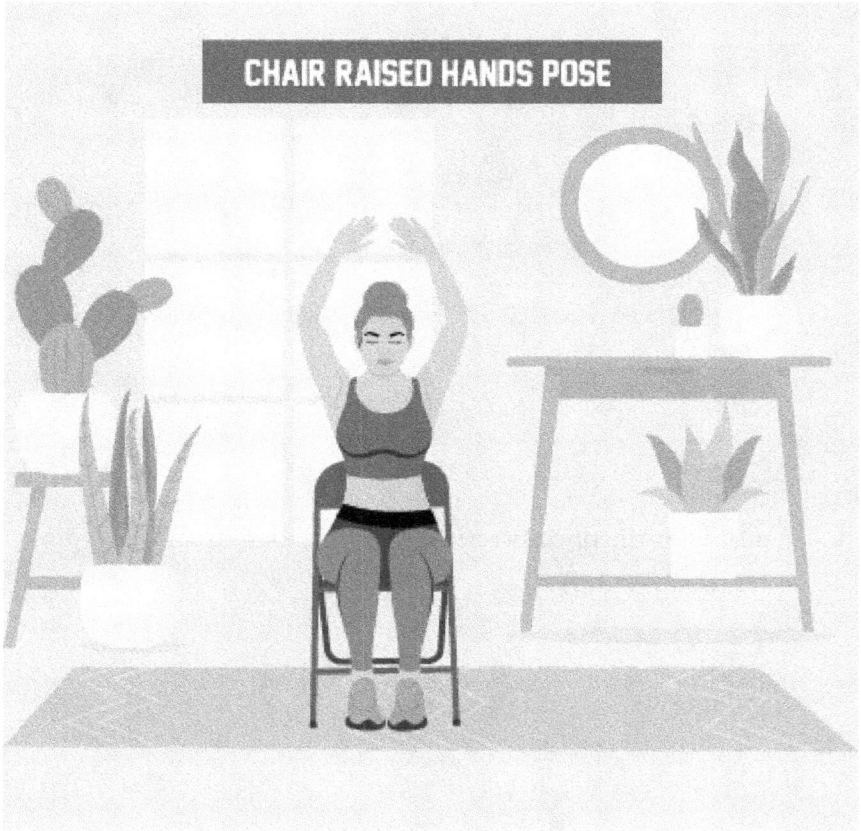

CHAIR RAISED HANDS POSE

5.4 Seated Five-Pointed Star

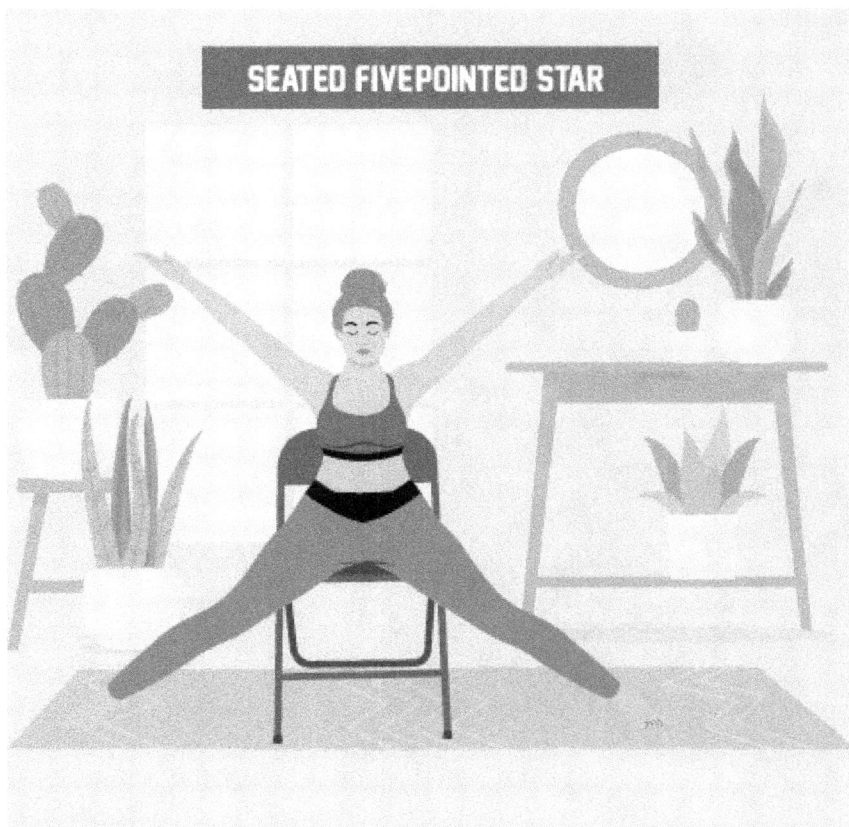

This pose strengthens, elongates, and aligns your spine as you wish upon a star. You can try it as:

1. Breathe deeply and spread your arms to either side. Do not tense up your spine. Your fingers and the top of your skull should expand.

2. Legs should be extended as straight as possible. Your head and limbs should work together to make the star that you are.

3. Hold for five breaths.

5.5 Crescent Lunge

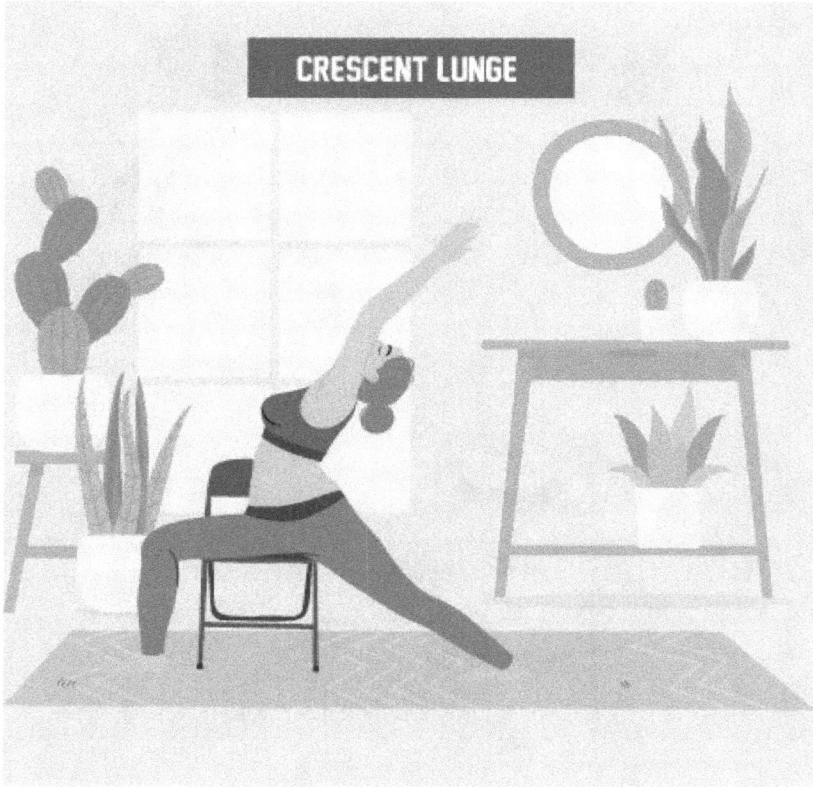

This pelvic tilt enables a deeper stretch of the psoas muscle and hip flexors. Below are instructions for you:

1. Lunge forward while keeping your thighs parallel and your front knee at a 90-degree angle.

2. Your feet should be separated from your shoulders.

3. Put pressure on the back leg's heel. Make sure not to elevate your shoulders when raising your arms above your head.

4. Up until you feel the lower back stretch and your abs draw in, slightly tuck the tailbone in to flatten down the front of the hips.

5. Hold for 20 breaths.

5.6 Hip Marches

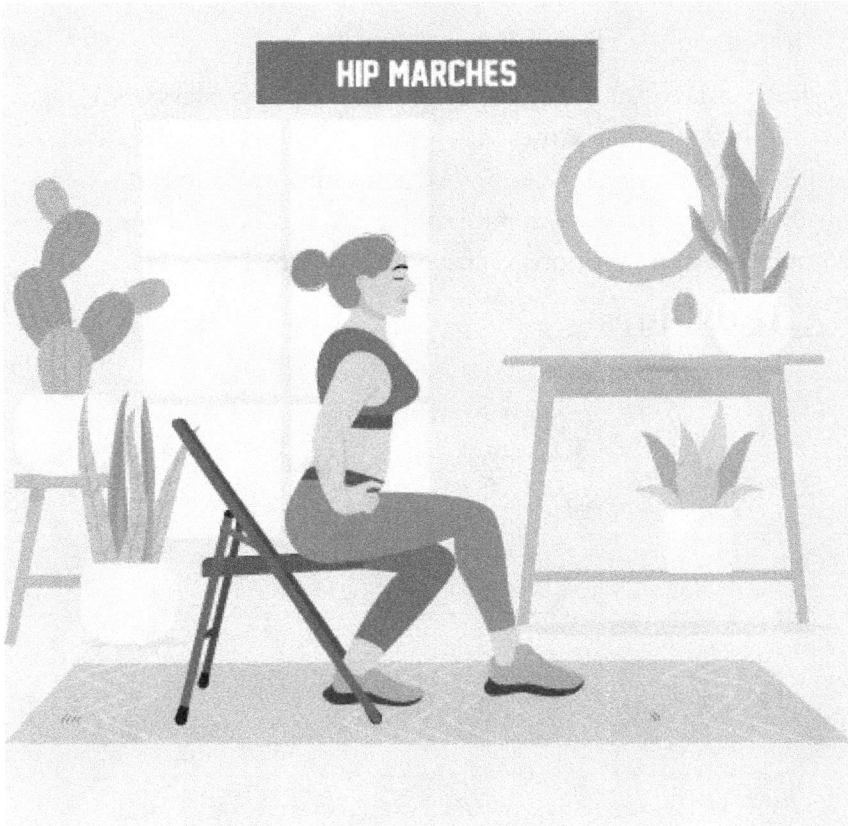

Sitting hip marches are a fantastic option for people who need to increase their hip flexibility and mobility or who want a modified way to do cardiovascular training. With the help of the following instructions, you can complete this exercise.

1. Place your feet firmly on the ground, hip distance apart, and sit tall in a strong chair.

2. To help maintain a tall posture, grab the chair's armrests or edges with both hands. At the same time, you need to contract your abdominal muscles.

3. As high as you can comfortably lift your right leg with the knee

bent as if performing a high-knee march.

4.   With control, bring your right foot to the ground.

5.   Repeat on the other side.

Perform at least 20 marches back-and-forth in succession. Repeat two or three more times after pausing. This exercise can be prolonged for a greater cardiovascular effect or added to a warm-up to help increase heart rate and get the blood flowing before completing more motions focused on strength.

5.7 Heal Slides

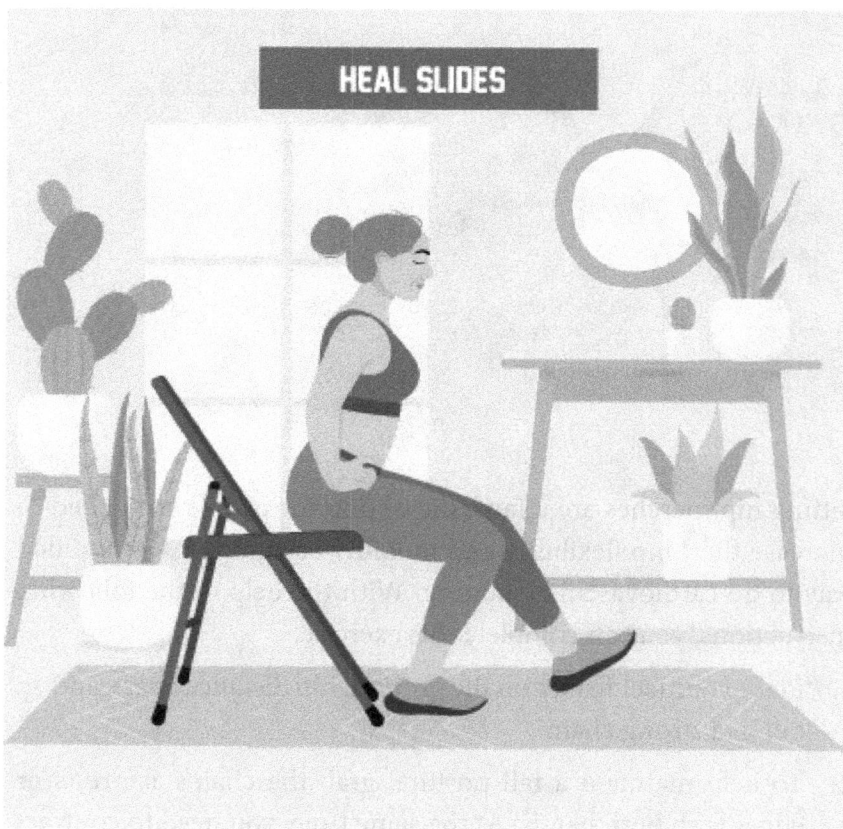

You need to do this pose with 3 Sets where one set has 8-10 reps. This flexibility yoga pose goes like this:

1. Keep your chest out, your abs firm, and both hands on the edge of the chair for stability while you sit comfortably at the edge of the chair.

2. Next, extend one leg forward while maintaining the other naturally bent, toes pointing forward.

3. Draw the extended foot backwards gradually while keeping its sole level on the ground until it is back in its original position.

4. Repeat the movement with the other leg.

5.8 Captain's Chair

Your abs and other core muscles will get stronger from this workout. You need to do this pose with 3 Sets where one set has 8-10 reps. It goes like this:

1. Make sure the chair is solid. Straighten your back out and hold onto the seat's sides.

2. Lift your feet off the ground gradually. Bringing your knees up to your chest.

3. At the top, tighten your abs, and then carefully descend your feet back to the ground.

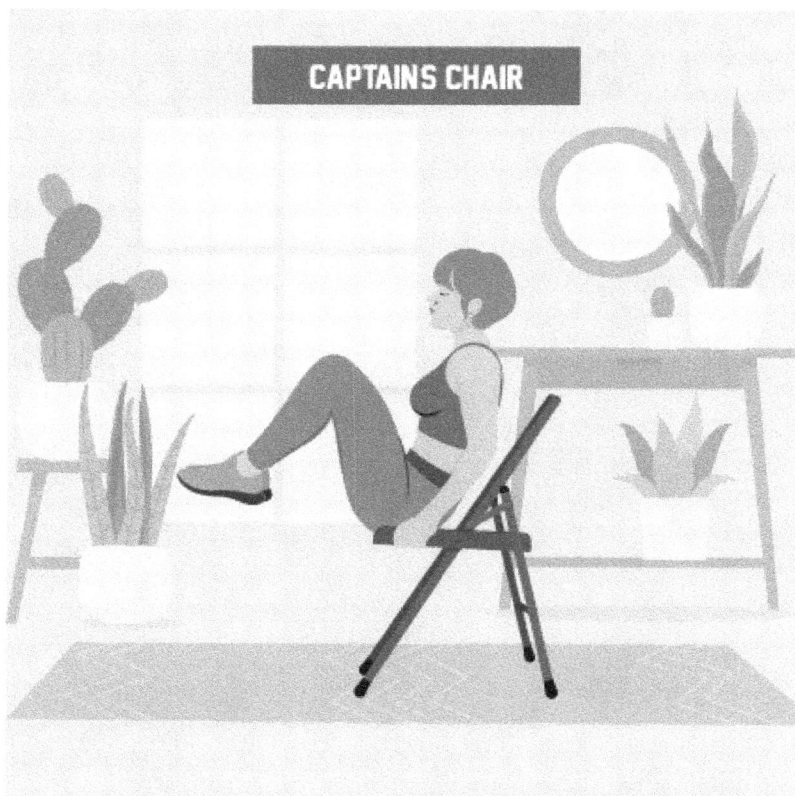

CAPTAINS CHAIR

Never attempt to move past a comfortable position. It is okay if you can only lift your feet a few inches off the ground.

5.9 Reverse Warrior

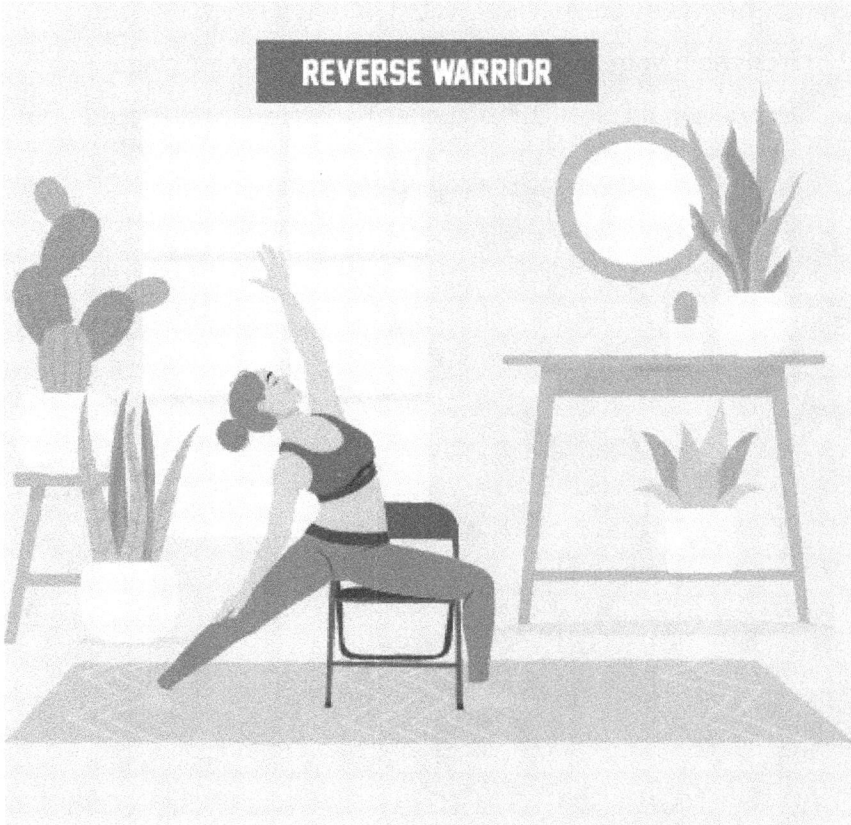

Follow the steps below for reverse warrior.

1. On an inhalation for the reverse warrior, let the left arm descend the left leg and raise the right arm to the ceiling.

2. Hold for three breaths.

3. Before sitting sideways on the chair facing left and performing the series of three warrior postures on the left side, bring both legs to the front of the chair.

5.10 Seated Jumping Jacks

Here is how you can go about seated jumping jacks.

1. Straighten your spine and sit on the edge of your chair.

2. As you would do with a standard jumping jack, extend your

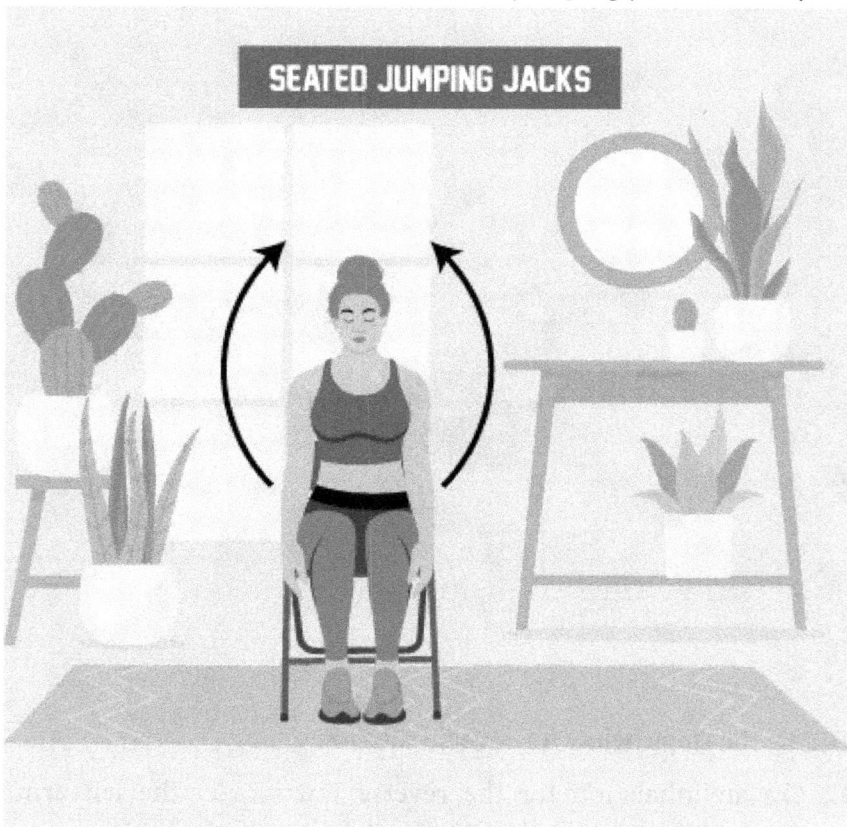

SEATED JUMPING JACKS

arms out to the sides and then up above your head.

3. Before raising your arms once more, place them back at your

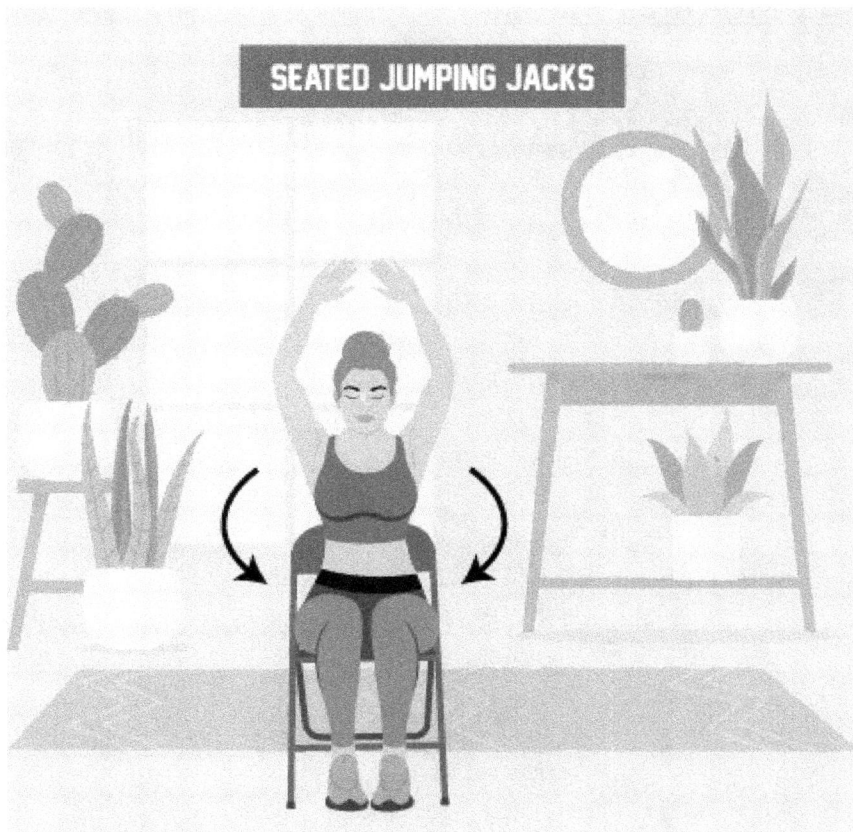

SEATED JUMPING JACKS

sides.

4. Start off slowly, and then pick up the pace until you can move your arms as quickly as you can.

5. Perform as many repetitions as you can.

6. Be careful not to hit the armrests while moving when exercising on a chair with arms.

5.11 Modified Planks

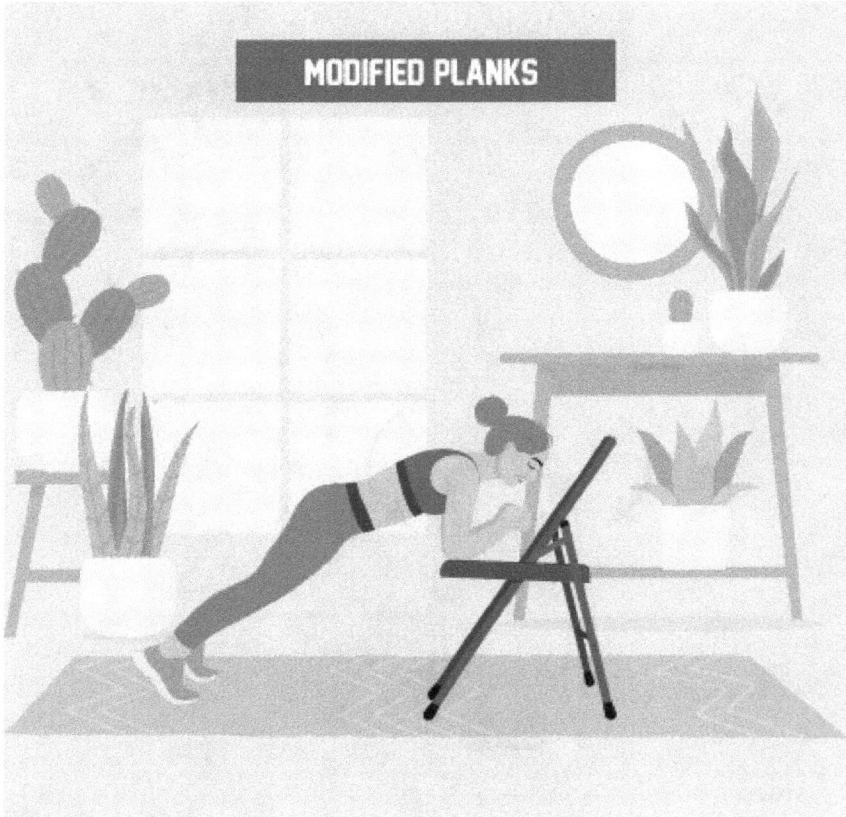

The entire front part of the body gains strength and stability during planks. It can be too difficult to maintain your entire body weight. Fortunately, the exercise can be accessible with a quick chair modification.

1. To ensure stability and that it would not move while you are completing the plank, place the chair in front of a wall.

2. You can either position the chair so that the seat faces the wall and you have access to the chair's back for support, or you can position it so that the back faces the wall and you have access to the chair's seat for support.

3. Adults who are less mobile or strong should begin by using the chair's back as support.

4. Once the chair is securely affixed to the wall, position your hands shoulder distance apart on the chair's back (or seat, depending on the chair's position).

5. Step backwards while contracting your abs until a straight diagonal line runs from your heels to the top of your head.

6. You should feel your abdominals trying to maintain the stability of your body as your arms and hips should be precisely straight and positioned between your knees and shoulders, respectively.

7. After holding the position for 10 to 60 seconds, rise up again.

8. Complete three sets of each plank, holding it for as long as you can while keeping your form intact.

5.12 Chair Running

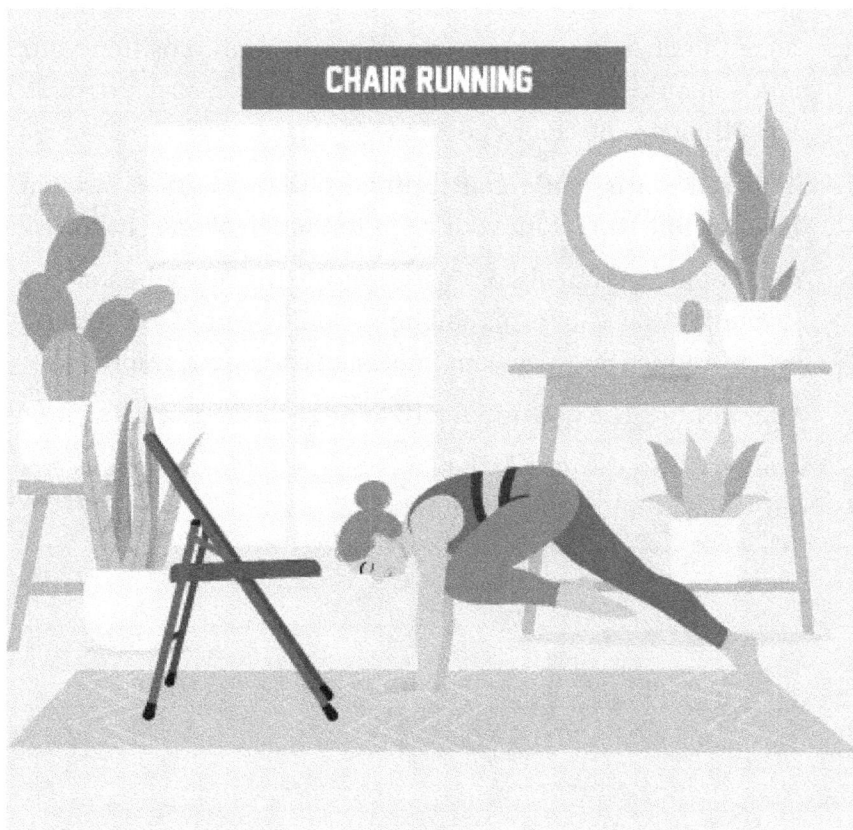

You need to do this pose with 3 Sets where one set has 8-10 reps. Follow the steps below for chair running:

1. Your arms should be at your sides. Your legs should be straight.

2. Adjust your posture in a way that your shoulder blades barely reach the chair's back.

3. Lift your feet up slowly off the ground.

4. Pull one knee towards you while keeping the other extended similar to running action.

5. If required, hold onto your seat's sides or armrests to maintain balance.

5.13 Ankle Rotations

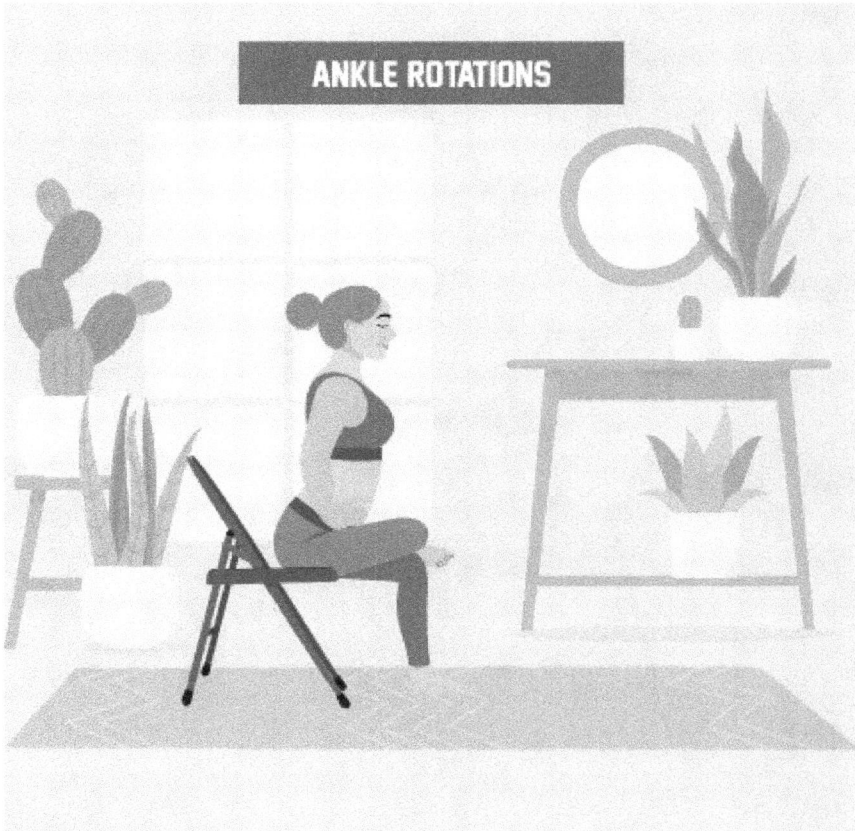

Repeat this exercise with 3 Sets where one set has 8-10 reps. Follow the steps below for ankle rotations:

1. Place your ankle on the knee to the opposite and sit up straight.

2. Swing your ankle around.

3. Make ten clockwise and ten counterclockwise rotations.

4. Stretch out even further by pointing your toes.

5.14 Sit and Reach

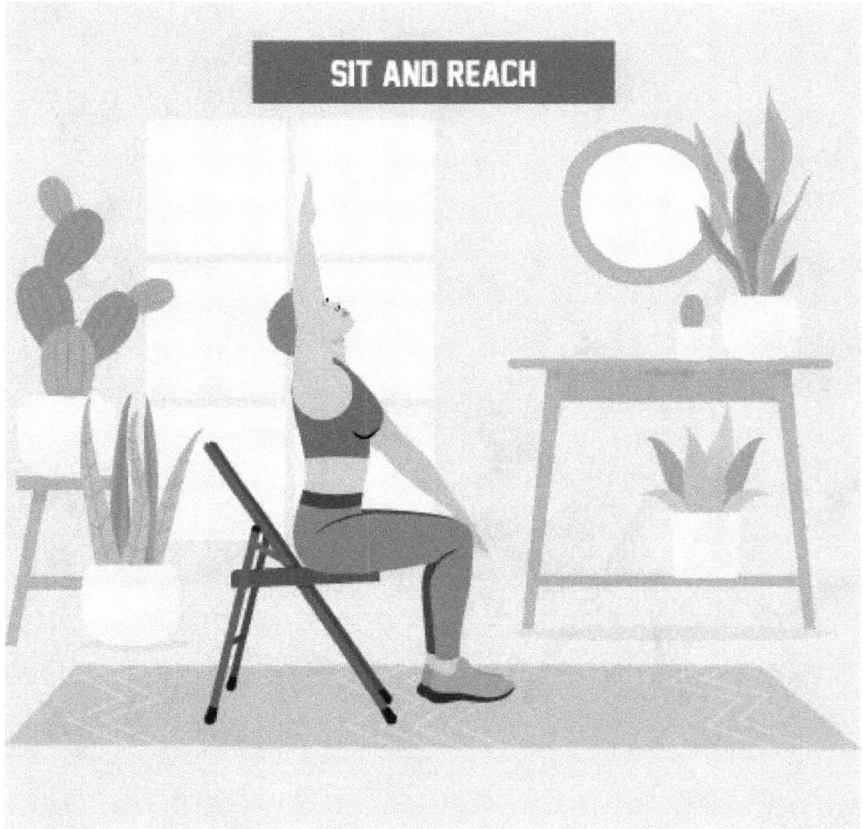

Reaching down to tie your shoe or extending to the top shelf both feel better when you are flexible and have a full range of motion. Flexibility makes it easier to move around and carry out daily tasks by reducing stiffness and soreness. You can follow the steps below:

1. Knees should be touching, and your back should be straight.

2. One arm should be extended straight up in the air.

3. Feel the strain as you raise your body and extend your torso.

4. To stretch your neck and shoulders, look in the direction of your hand.

5. After holding the position for five to ten seconds, switch to the opposite side.

6. Repeat three times per side.

5.15 Leg Lifts

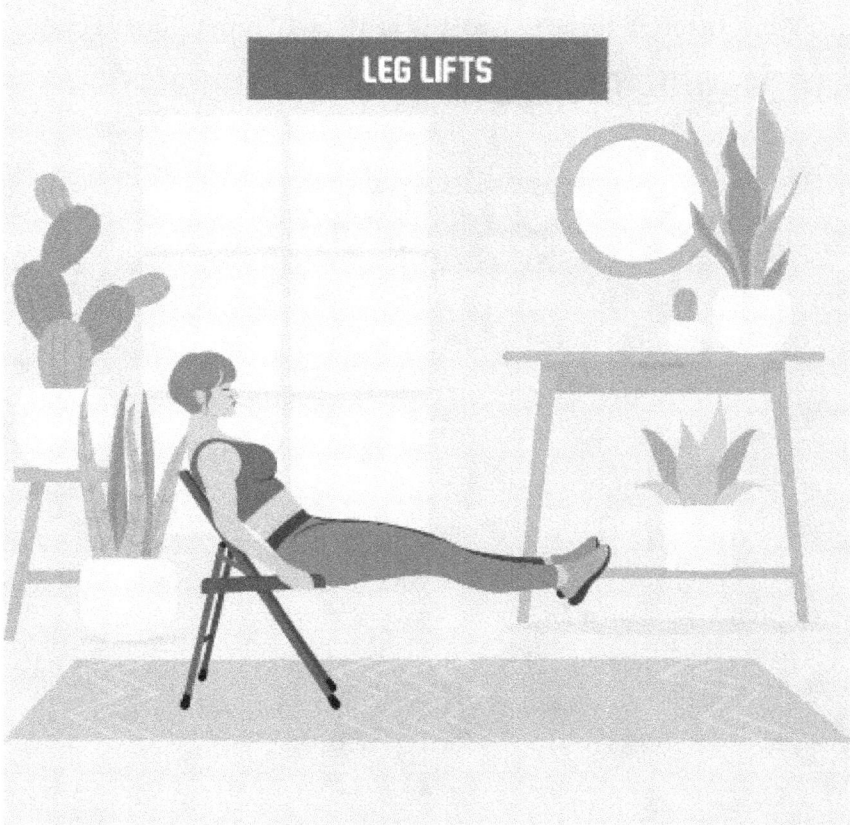

You may strengthen your core by performing a chair-based modified leg raise. Although it is ideal to do this exercise in a firm chair with armrests, you can also do it while clutching the chair's edges next to your hips.

1. Sit up straight in a chair with your feet flat on the floor and your core engaged.

2. To maintain proper posture, roll your shoulders back.

3. Hold onto the armrests or seat of the chair. As you exhale, elevate both legs as high as you can (knees bent) while keeping your feet and knees together.

4. After holding for 5 seconds, bring your feet back down to the ground.

5. Work through three to five sets of 10 to 12 repetitions each.

5.16 Modified Burpees

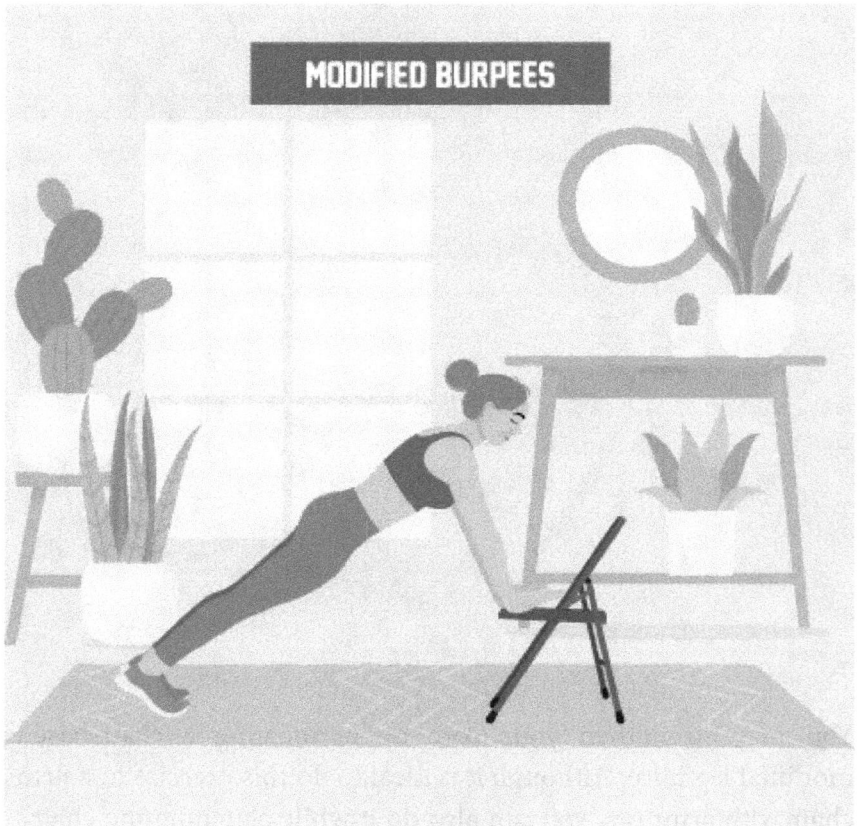

Older folks might not be able to perform strict burpees, but with changes, they might be completely safe depending on strength and mobility. For example, try performing a burpee as follows:

1. To prevent the chair from sliding or moving, push it up against

a wall with the back against the wall.

2. Standing with your feet roughly shoulder-width apart, face the chair.

3. To get into a half-squat position, push your hips back and flex your knees.

4. With your arms fully extended and palms facing inward, firmly place both hands on the chair's seat.

5. Step one foot back, then the other, forming a modified chair plank position with your body aligned straight from heel to head.

6. Reverse the motion, then advance each foot to the beginning position.

7. As you stand up, lengthen your hips and knees while pressing through your feet. Clap your hands together while raising your arms above your head.

This is equivalent to one modified chair burpee. Try to complete as many (six to ten) in perfect form as you can. Complete at least two or three sets.

5.17 Small Kicks

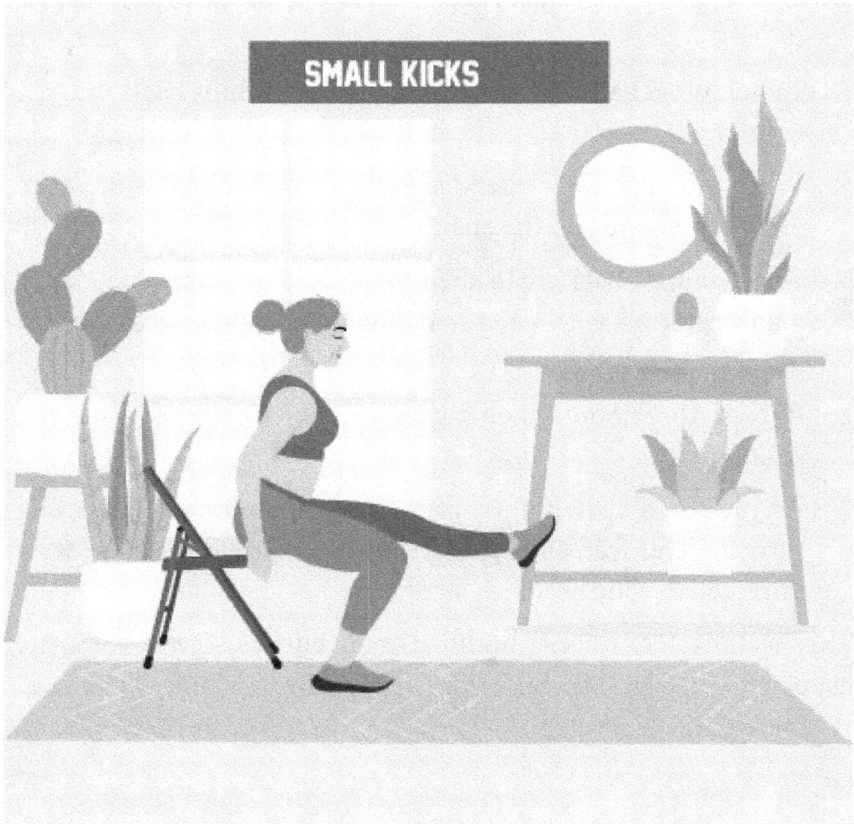

Small kicks resemble knee extensions in several ways but are faster. You will move more like you are kicking to get those muscles going rather than pausing in the middle! These are the steps for small kicks.

1. Sit on just the edge of your chair with your hands on the side for further support. Keep your knees bent and your feet flat on the ground.

2. Quickly extend your right knee and lift your right foot as if you were kicking a ball.

3. After kicking, bring the foot back to the ground.

4. Switch to your left leg.

5. Do 15 to 20 repetitions per leg.

5.18 Chair Squats

Here is how you can go about chair squats:

1. Sit in a chair with your arms by your sides and your back

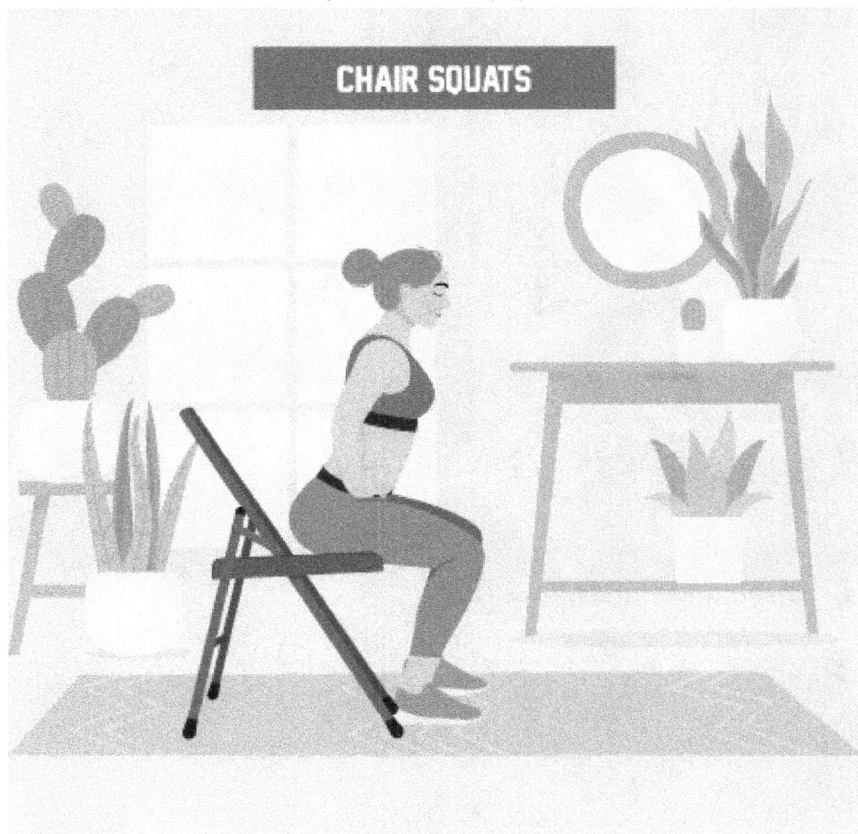

    straight.

2. As you stand tall, press your heels and the middle of your feet into the ground. Keep your chest upright at all times.

3. Once you have sat back down on the chair, lower yourself into a squat position by bending at the hips, pulling your hips back, and bending your knees.

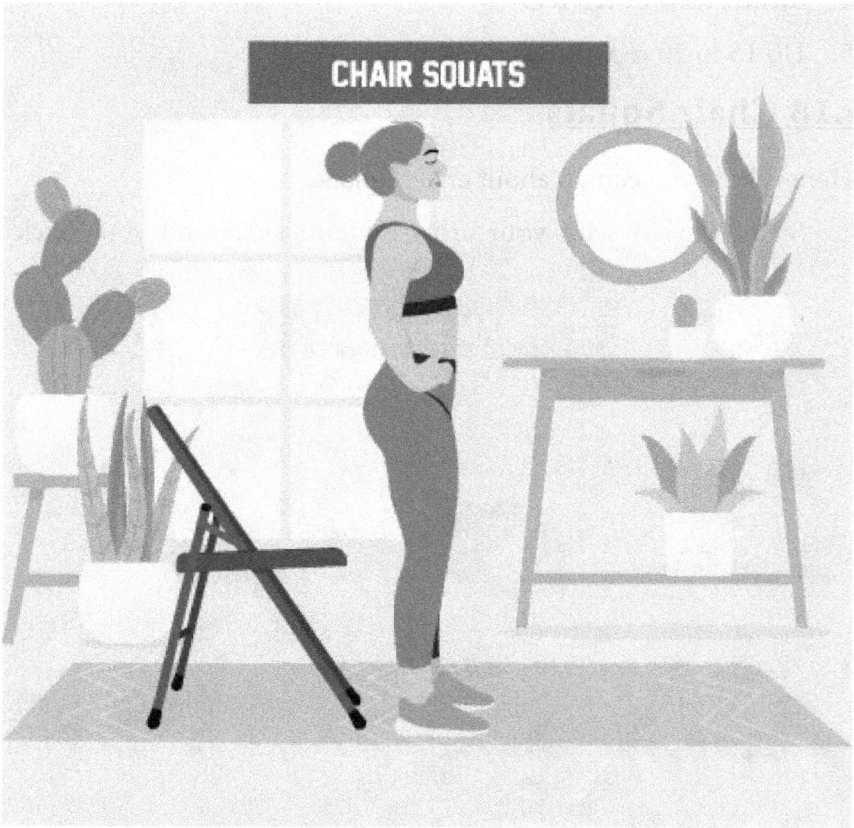

CHAIR SQUATS

4. Do ten repetitions.

5.19 Calf Stretch

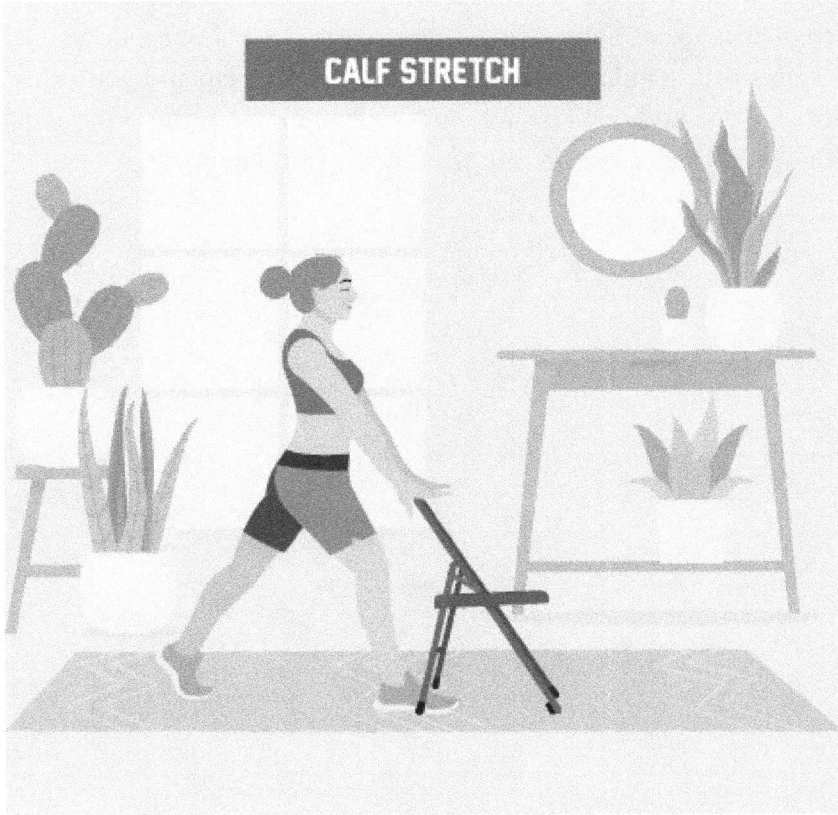

You can stretch your calf muscles by performing these exercises for seniors in a standing chair. You need to:

1. Face the chair's back from approximately an arm's length away.

2. For support, place your hands on the chair's back.

3. Step back with your right foot, pointing both of your feet in the direction of the chair.

4. Keep your right heel planted to the ground as you lean forward.

5. Hold for 30 seconds with three repetitions.

6. Switching sides and repeat the instructions.

These poses will help you improve your mobility and flexibility. When you are done practicing your daily exercises, spend a few minutes sitting quietly with your hands on your lap and your eyes closed. Your body will be able to fully benefit from the poses you just did as you transition into the rest of your day.

Conclusion

An active lifestyle has many well-known and proven advantages. Exercise is the best medicine, as it is often claimed. Fortunately, everyone can benefit from and participate in chair yoga. As a safer and more pleasant approach to practicing yoga despite having reduced mobility, lower fitness levels, sight or balance impairments, and weakness, chair yoga has evolved into a therapeutic movement practice that is specifically geared toward seniors or older individuals.

You will start to feel a sense of peace and relaxation flow through your body once you start doing chair yoga. You will gradually notice that the tension that formerly engulfed your muscles and joints starts dissipating, making it easy to perform routine everyday duties.

Seniors, especially those with significant mobility limitations, can choose chair yoga as an easy and practical workout. These exercises can be modified for individual mobility restrictions and gradually become more difficult. The body will receive more oxygen with the aid of chair yoga, and the brain, heart, fingers, and toes will all regenerate. Numerous breathing techniques can help you relax and are especially beneficial if you have mobility concerns.

Yoga activities, including breathing exercises, can be performed at any time, inside and outside the home, using a moderate approach. You can benefit from the many advantages of yoga, including improved circulation, a sense of well-being, and reductions in blood pressure, anxiety, inflammation, anxiety, and chronic pain, by using your chair for seated poses or balanced poses.

This graphical book focuses on chair yoga postures specifically for seniors to improve mobility, back pain, posture and balance. The book's first chapter provides a crash course on chair yoga, defining the benefits and ways to customize yoga poses for your needs, along with an exercise plan. The chapter ends with breathing exercises to help you set the tone for your relaxing yoga journey.

The next four chapters include step-by-step instructions with illustrations on yoga poses for balance, stability, posture, muscle strain, back pain, body strength, flexibility and mobility, e.g. seated mountain pose, moving crescent moon, foot to seat pose, chair hip extensions, clock reach, thread the needle, roll-downs, cobra chair pose etc.

If you have found this yoga book helpful, please leave a review on Amazon.

www.ingramcontent.com/pod-product-compliance
Lightning Source LLC
Chambersburg PA
CBHW060245030426
42335CB00014B/1605